Prostate Tales

*Men's Experiences
with Prostate Cancer*

Other books by Ross Gray, Ph.D.

Legacy: A Conversation with Dad
(with Claire Gray; Men's Studies Press, 2001)

*Standing Ovation: Performing Social Science
Research About Cancer*
(with C. Sinding; Altamira Press, 2002)

Prostate Tales

Men's Experiences
with Prostate Cancer

Ross Gray, Ph.D.

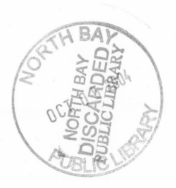

Men's Studies Press, Harriman, Tennessee 37748
Copyright 2003 by the Men's Studies Press, LLC.

Book Team
Executive editor: James Doyle
Developmental editor: Suzin Seaton
Cover and text design: Sally Ham Govan
Production manager: David Prentice
Cover photo © Digital Vision

First Edition
ISBN: 1-931342-00-8

Library of Congress Cataloging-in-Publication Data

Gray, Ross E.
    Prostate tales: men's experiences with prostate cancer / by Ross
        Gray.—1st ed. p. cm.
    Includes bibliographical references.
    ISBN 1-93132-00-8 (pbk.: alk. paper) – ISBN 1-931342-01-6
        (e-version)
    1. Prostate—Cancer—Psychological aspects.
    2. Prostate— Cancer—Social aspects.
    I. Title.
RC280.P7 .G73 2002
616.99'463'0019—dc21

                                            2002006995

Contents

Acknowledgment   i

Foreword by Wally Seeley   iii

Prologue   1

Roger Discovers His Prostate   5
    Men's Health Attitudes and Practices   16

I'll Sail Away   19
    About Masculinity   24

Maurice Runs a Meeting   27
    Men Helping Men?   38

Carl Retreats to the Den   41
    Relationships with Spouses   49

Jed Meets Brad and Steven   51
    Men and Diversity   60

Ben Answers the Phone   61
    Making Treatment Decisions   66

John Takes a Walk   69
    Recovering from Treatment   75

Frederick Tries for a Job   77
   Urinary Incontinence   82

Norm Downs a Few Drinks   85
   Erectile Dysfunction (Impotence)   90

Doug Goes Fishing   95
   Prostate Cancer and Depression   100

I Was Just a Number   103
   Work and Insurance Issues   107

Simon Cultivates Romance   111
   Metastatic Disease and Hormone Treatments   119

Darren Celebrates a Birthday   121
   Hormone Refractory Disease and Palliative Care   126

No Big Deal? by Vrenia Ivonoffski and Ross Gray   129
   Research-Based Theatre   171

Appendix A—Prostate Cancer Basics   173

Appendix B—Reflections on the Writing of *Prostate Tales*:
   Locating the Work within Personal and Academic
   Contexts   177

Glossary   185

Resources   191

Acknowledgment

I want to acknowledge the important contributions to this work by team members Margaret Fitch, Karen Fergus, Kathryn Church, and Eric Mykhalovskiy, in our study of prostate cancer and masculinity, funded by the Canadian Institutes of Health Research. I also want to record my debt to friends and colleagues who have supported me along the way, said encouraging things, helped me to believe I might finish the manuscript, and suggested that it would be worth the effort. Thanks, then, to Chris Sinding, Terry Mitchell, Judy Gould, Fran Turner, Ralph Osborne, Andrew Sparkes, Ken Gray, Dawn Lawrick, and Paul Soren. Let me also express my gratitude to Vrenia Ivonoffski, co-writer of *No Big Deal?*, a great supporter, and a wonderful writing partner and teacher. Special thanks to Kathryn Church, who has shown me through her own brilliant example about the value of taking risks and crossing academic boundaries, and who has encouraged my writer's spirit every step of the way.

I feel privileged to be connected to the Men's Studies Press, and especially grateful for the generous support of James Doyle. This book would not have happened without his enthusiastic encouragement. I also want to thank Suzin Seaton for engaging so passionately with the manuscript and for her capable assistance in developing and refining it.

I also want to acknowledge and thank the men with prostate cancer who agreed to participate, and who shared much of themselves. A special thanks is due to the leaders of the prostate cancer patient movement for doing such important work on behalf of ill men.

Foreword

Recently I was in New York City attending a seminar and had the opportunity to visit Cancer Care New York. Established in 1943, this organization has a well-adjudicated array of publications to help cancer patients. As I glanced through this impressive collection, I noticed a brochure produced by the Cancer Hope Network in New Jersey entitled "CANCER? Get Past the Diagnosis—Talk to Someone Who's Been There." The two-page brochure described the information and comfort one could receive from Cancer Hope. Not only did this brochure describe a prime reason for prostate cancer support groups, but also one of the purposes of this excellent book.

This year 180,000 American men and nearly 18,000 Canadian men will be told they have prostate cancer. Although the mortality rate of prostate cancer is slowly coming down due primarily to early detection, there continues to be a veritable explosion in the number of men being diagnosed with this disease. Each of these men has had to cope with the statement, "You have prostate cancer." Once the initial anger, denial, and remorse are dealt with, support beyond the professional level is usually sought. Often a survivor friend or local support group is approached. *Prostate Tales* is a valuable addition to these excellent resources.

For the many whose cancer is beyond the prostate gland, *Prostate Tales* can help by showing how other men have coped with incontinence, impotence, and other side effects. Through the experiences described in these stories, *Prostate Tales* addresses most of the questions a man and his family face as they cope with this disease.

Prostate Tales as well gives the treatment professional a glimpse of the patient side of the equation. Often the pressures of practice do not allow a treatment specialist the time to discuss the emotional aspects of this cancer with a patient. The layout of *Prostate Tales* enables the reader to zero in on a difficulty or troublesome subject without having to read the book from page one. Superbly referenced with a useful glossary, it becomes a reference manual as well as a good read.

Prostate cancer is a silent killer. In its curable state it has no symptoms. *Prostate Tales* will be an invaluable aid to men interested in finding out more about prostate cancer, and for those diagnosed with the disease, it's like having a support group on the night table beside your bed.

WALLY SEELEY
Executive Director
Canadian Prostate Cancer Network
Lakefield, Ontario
July 2002

Prologue

This is a book about men with prostate cancer and the people who care about them. It's about their crises, their struggles, their sorrows, their challenges, and their triumphs. It's about how prostate cancer disrupts and changes men's lives.

My intention in writing *Prostate Tales* has been to bring the experiences of men with prostate cancer to life, to pull them out of the shadows where they usually lie, to make men's lives bright and vivid. *Prostate Tales* will be particularly relevant for men with prostate cancer, and for their spouses and other family members and friends, but it will also be useful for health professionals, educators, and researchers.

Prostate cancer directly affects one in eight men in the Western world. It indirectly affects many more people, including spouses, children, friends, and co-workers. While prostate cancer is, after lung cancer, the most common cause of cancer-related death among men, some men are cancer-free after treatment, and others live with the disease for many years. Many men eventually die of other disorders. The result of this situation is that most men diagnosed with prostate cancer face years of dealing with the challenging effects of disease and treatment.

I'm a social scientist working in a cancer program, and my impulse to do this writing came from my research with men who have prostate cancer. But *Prostate Tales* isn't much like many research reports that are written. For this book, I've turned away from the dry explanatory formulations of academic writing to write narrative accounts and create dramatic scripts. All of the accounts (except the last) are based on interviews our research team (Ross Gray, Margaret Fitch, Karen Fergus, Eric Mykhalovskiy, and Kathryn Church) conducted with men with prostate cancer in a study funded by the

Canadian Institutes for Health Research. Each man was interviewed four or five times. We asked the men about their experiences with prostate cancer and, beyond that, about their entire lives. In discussion with these men, we considered the full impact of prostate cancer.

The life situations described in the narrative accounts that follow were inspired by these interviews. Many of the words spoken by characters in the accounts were drawn directly from what men actually said in interviews. One part of my task in writing has been to honor the perspectives and expressions of the men we interviewed. Another part has been to protect their individual identities by fictionalizing their accounts, combining bits provided by various men and disguising identifying details.

The idea for *Prostate Tales* grew over time as I tried, through my research, to understand what men go through when they have prostate cancer. In one early study, I interviewed a man who had been a driving force in the formation of Canadian prostate cancer support groups. He commented, "There's not a lot of interest in, or sympathy for, sick old guys." Over the years, I kept returning to his words, wondering why I myself had taken so long to attend to the issues of men with cancer, wondering why colleagues showed little or no interest in my work with ill men, wondering why a nurse even ridiculed the men in a local support group. Bottom line, I became curious about why ill men were perceived as uninteresting.

Later, I surveyed men with prostate cancer across Canada, wanting to make sure that their needs and issues would be front and center at the first National Prostate Cancer Forum. Survey findings were intriguing. Although many men acknowledged problems as a result of cancer disease and treatment, most denied that prostate cancer negatively affected the quality of their lives. So, at least on the surface of things, men seemed to be doing just fine. Yet many men also wrote other kinds of messages in the spaces where we asked them to comment. One man wrote he felt like a neutered dog. Another admitted he had trouble thinking about his impotence without feeling bitter. Another was angry that doctors treated him like an idiot. But the one statement that most affected me was the following:

> Of course my diagnosis has changed my life. How can you really explain the pain, the anger, the tears, the loss of sex life after my operation. Although I don't have a sex life and I don't have a life free from fear or anger, I do have a life. I have a wife that loves me, I have a devoted child and wonderful grandchildren, a career that has given me income, pride, and challenge. I am a lucky man.

This was a man who had filled out his questionnaire to show that his quality of life had actually improved because of prostate cancer. I realized that many men were, indeed, grateful to be alive and to have received treatment, but that this in no way meant they did not suffer. On the contrary, in reading those comments on the questionnaires I started to understand a bit about what men really went through. And I started to look for better ways to communicate what I was learning—a search that eventually led me to write *Prostate Tales*.

How to Read *Prostate Tales*

Men (and those who care about them) often lack the kind of experiential information embedded in *Prostate Tales*, having to rely instead entirely on disembodied "facts" and statistics. While *Prostate Tales* does include some such facts, the book is not intended to provide a thorough detailing of prostate cancer information. Fortunately, there are now many high quality books and Internet sites available. *Prostate Tales* provides signposts about how to find some of these.

For a brief overview of medical issues, readers should refer to "Prostate Cancer Basics" in Appendix A at the end of the book. Informational essays following the accounts focus on issues featured in the accounts and list additional books and papers that might be helpful.

The primary audience for *Prostate Tales* is men who have been diagnosed with and treated for prostate cancer. In the accounts that follow, the reader will recognize familiar dilemmas related to cancer and see how other men have attempted to deal with the same dilemmas. *Prostate Tales* will be useful for men who are at risk of prostate cancer, or who have been recently diagnosed, because it provides accessible information about the implications of various treatment choices and reveals the landscapes of men's illness experiences. *Prostate Tales* will also be useful for spouses (and other family members and friends) who want to better understand what their men are going through. The book provides insights into how to be helpful to ill men and provides starting points for important family discussions. Some of these insights are equally relevant for health professionals engaged in caring for men with prostate cancer. Finally, anyone interested in innovative approaches to education and the communication of research findings should find *Prostate Tales* an intriguing model.

The accounts in *Prostate Tales* reveal the pathways different men take in facing prostate cancer. In some of the accounts, characters speak strongly for a particular medical approach. For example, in "Ben Answers the Phone," Larry is relentless in his promotion of surgery as the best way of treating prostate cancer. But in another story, "Carl Retreats to the Den," a man in different life circumstances argues differently, preferring radiation treatment. I am not selling any particular point of view, simply showing how various men travel through the maze of medical uncertainty to come to decisions.

In Appendix B, I argue for new approaches to communicating research findings, including narrative accounts and dramas like those found in *Prostate Tales*. There is now a growing awareness among researchers of the need to disseminate information in ways that are useful to people. And more social scientists are experimenting with innovative approaches to writing. Appendix B locates *Prostate Tales* within a rapidly evolving academic movement.

If you have feedback about *Prostate Tales*, please send it to me at ross.gray@tsrcc.on.ca.

Roger Discovers His Prostate

Roger is a 54-year-old white man, about to be diagnosed with prostate cancer, eventually to have a radical prostatectomy. He is married and is employed as a business executive.

Doctor Garshowitz

Roger glances at his watch, is startled to see it's already past 3 p.m. He rolls back from his desk, pushes to his feet. He has a sudden impulse to cancel the appointment but he knows that he'd just have to re-book it. The company has been clamping down for a few years now, making sure that managers go for their check-ups. It's a waste of time as far as he's concerned, but he's not going to make any more waves about it. Better to save himself for bigger battles.

The company doctor has his office four floors up, so Roger ambles in the direction of the elevators. He may have to do it, but he'll be damned if he's going to rush to get there, late or not. Last year he complained to the doctor that check-ups are like taking your car to a garage. You always find that something is wrong, but that doesn't necessarily mean it needs to be fixed. Only a few of Roger's friends go for regular medical exams, and that's either because their wives harass them, or because, like Roger, they have company plans.

He nods and says hello to people in the elevator. Everybody knows him. Which is about what you'd expect after 30 years, working his way up, one step at a time, from the mailroom right through to management. On the 11th floor, he walks to the end of the hall, knocks once, and pushes the door open. Dr. Garshowitz, a short, thin man in his 60s, leans against the far wall.

"You're late." He glances at his watch.

"Oh, well, I'm here."

"Men your age need to be pay attention to their health." The doctor's smiling, but clearly means what he says.

"Yeah. Sure." Roger doesn't need the pep talk. He's heard it all before.

The doctor asks him a series of questions. Roger explains himself. Sure, he's a few pounds up from the last time, but that's no big deal. And he doesn't get to the gym very often. But he has a busy work and family life, and you can't do everything you'd like to do. And yes, he's still smoking a half-pack a day. The doctor raises his eyebrows at that, but Roger glares at him, making it clear that the subject isn't open for discussion.

"Go into the examining room, take all your clothes off, and put the gown on with the opening at the back. I'll be right with you."

"Right." Roger's thinking about the presentation he has to make at the marketing meeting this afternoon. He just wants to get this over with.

Dr. Garshowitz makes him cough several times, hits his knee with a hammer, listens to his heart, does the blood pressure thing. But then there's something different.

"I need you to bend over because I want to give you a rectal exam. At your age, we need to start watching your prostate."

Roger is confused. He's not sure he knows what a prostate is. And he doesn't like the sound of this exam.

"Are you sure this is necessary?"

"Trust me. A lot of guys your age get prostate problems, and it's good to find out early if that's happening." The doctor's pulling on a plastic glove. "What I'm going to do is insert my finger in your rectum and feel the prostate to see whether it's normal."

"Listen, I haven't been having any problems. I don't think we need to worry."

Dr. Garshowitz stops pulling at the glove and looks at Roger directly. "This is part of your annual medical check-up. Why don't you just bend over, and it'll be over in a second."

Roger groans and complies. "Whatever you feel you need to do."

It doesn't exactly hurt, but it's awfully uncomfortable, and he's panicked by the intrusion. When he straightens up again, Roger feels disoriented. He grabs the chair next to him, sits heavily.

"If you're feeling dizzy just put your head down for a minute. Sometimes that happens." The doctor is sounding sympathetic now. Roger feels stupid to be reacting like this, but he puts his head down anyway.

"We'll need to keep an eye on your prostate. It feels like there might be a bit of swelling on one side. I'm going to get your PSA done when you go for blood."

Roger doesn't know what a PSA is. Right now, he doesn't care. "So can I go?"

"Yes. Here's the order for the lab work. Try and get there today or tomorrow."

"Sure." He has no intention of going today. Maybe he'll fit it in next week sometime. Roger doesn't like needles. And, besides, he has more important things to do.

"See you next year."

"Ok. I'll call if there are any problems with the lab work, but I'm sure it'll be fine. And try and cut down on the cigarettes."

Roger bangs the door after him. Bloody doctors can never resist having the last word.

Doctor Martindale—Eight months later

Roger sits in the waiting room, trying not to cough because once he starts it's hard to stop. He's been hacking away for weeks now, and when he finally went to see about a prescription from Dr. Garshowitz, wouldn't you know he was off on vacation somewhere in the Caribbean. Doctors! Roger would have given up at that point, but his wife Sarah suggested he see her family doctor. So here he is, copy of his medical file from work in hand.

Dr. Martindale is a stocky 40ish man with a friendly, pragmatic approach. Roger likes him right away, likes how he diagnoses the lung problem quickly, how he gives exactly the right amount of information about taking the antibiotic. After writing the prescription, Dr. Martindale asks Roger if he's having any other problems, flipping through Roger's chart while he's waiting for an answer.

Roger says no, he's fine otherwise. But then he notices the doctor frowning.

"I see that your PSA level was a bit high at your last checkup."

Roger notes the concerned tone, but doesn't have a clue what the doctor is concerned about. "So what does a high PSA mean?"

"Well, it can indicate a prostate problem. It's not elevated a lot, but a level of 6 shouldn't be ignored. Have you had a biopsy?"

"No. But my company doctor never said anything about needing a biopsy." Roger doesn't like where this is heading.

"I think you should have one. Would you like me to arrange it, or would you like to arrange it through your company doctor?"

Roger isn't ready to give in yet. "Convince me why I should have a biopsy. I hate to put you on the spot, but I don't want to have things done to me without good reason."

The doctor is nonplussed. "There are various problems that can be associated with high PSA levels, and it's important to rule out that nothing serious is going on." He looks at Roger and sees that he's still unconvinced. "If you were my father, I'd have you in for a biopsy this afternoon."

The last statement gets to Roger, especially because the doctor delivers it with such sincerity. He capitulates.

"That's good enough for me. I think I'll go get a biopsy." Roger is amazed that he sounds so matter of fact, because inside his stomach's doing somersaults.

Dr. Martindale smiles. "Good. It's the sensible thing to do. If you want to just wait a few minutes, I'll make the arrangements and let you know what to do next."

Doctor Angrosino—Two weeks later

Roger isn't happy about being in the position he's in. Not happy at all. He didn't know what a biopsy would involve, but it's worse than he imagined. Dr. Angrosino, a big lanky guy younger than his son, told Roger that the instrument was like a pellet gun and that he would be taking some shots at his prostate.

When he was eight, Roger got hit in the back of the head by a pellet from his brother's rifle. He isn't reassured by the doctor's explanation.

He's been counting the "shots," and it's up to six. The doctor said he would be doing ten, so Roger's holding on, waiting for the end. Each shot is a bit more uncomfortable. The sense of pressure of the gun inside him is aggravating, scary. Roger counts to himself, seven, eight, nine. God, he wants out of here. And then, finally, ten. But something's wrong. The doctor doesn't seem to be done.

"Aren't you finished? You said ten."

"Oh, that was just a rough guess. I'm going to do a few more." Gives a little chuckle.

Roger sees nothing funny, exhales deeply. Eleven. Twelve. Thirteen. Oh, bloody hell. Fourteen.

"Okay. We're done."

Roger tries to relax. He's incredibly sore.

"So what exactly is this all about?"

The doctor looks surprised by the question. "Well, we're trying to find out if there's a tumor there."

Roger puts a hand on the examining table to steady himself. "So by that do you mean cancer?"

"That's right."

"Okay." He let's that sink in for a second. Then he shifts to thinking about a more immediate concern. "What am I supposed to do now? I can't sit down, and I don't see how I can walk."

The doctor smiles brightly. "That's normal. Go and have a coffee and rest for a while. You'll be okay in a couple of hours. If you have any complications, give me a call, but you should be fine. I'll be sending the biopsy results to your family doctor."

Roger takes a small step, winces, takes another. Says goodbye to Dr. Angrosino. Wishes the good doctor could feel what it's like, just for a minute. Maybe he wouldn't be so cheerful.

Doctor Martindale again—Three weeks later

Roger opens the front door, and Sarah is there within seconds. They hug and kiss. He always misses her desperately when he's away on business. Sarah watches while he hangs up his coat. Asks him about the flight from New York. Uneventful. He asks her about her day at work. Uneventful. It's good to be home. He's thinking he'll have a whiskey and watch the news. Sarah follows him to the kitchen.

"There's a message for you from Dr. Martindale."

Roger's hand freezes on the cupboard door. "Did he say what he wants?"

"Just for you to call him."

Roger doesn't reply. He pushes down the rising fear. It's probably nothing. He pulls out the bottle, pours a drink, then heads for the TV room.

The next day, Roger has a strategic planning marathon at work. It's only when he gets home, when Sarah asks, that he remembers he was supposed to call Dr. Martindale. He tells her he doesn't want to call, that he has too many things going on at work right now. She threatens him. Says if he doesn't call, she'll call for him. He relents. Promises to do it in the morning.

When Dr. Martindale comes to the phone the next morning, he asks Roger to come to his office right away. That scares Roger enough to cancel a meeting, get in his car, and drive across town. Now he's sitting across from Dr. Martindale, who's looking serious, meaty hands folded in front of him.

"Roger, the results from your biopsy have come back, and they're positive."

Roger stares at him. "They're positive? Well, that's good news, isn't it? I don't understand."

"By positive I mean they found something. I'm sorry to say that there's a tumor in your prostate."

Roger just stares. He can't think of anything to say. He's numb.

Dr. Martindale clears his throat. "So now you need to decide what you're going to do about the tumor."

Roger keeps staring, shakes his head to try and shake his mind free from its paralysis. "What do you mean what am I going to do about it? You're the doctor. Why don't you tell me what steps I need to take?"

The hands on the desk look less composed. Fingers from one hand tear at a cuticle on the other. The doctor looks grim.

"With prostate cancer it's not so straightforward. There are a number of possibilities. And I can't make the decision for you. You're going to have to make some inquiries. I'd suggest that you talk to a few prostate cancer specialists. Then we could meet again if you'd like and discuss what you've learned. The one thing you should know is that prostate cancer is usually slow-growing, so you don't have to rush into anything."

Later, Roger can't remember leaving the doctor's office, can't remember what he was supposed to do next. He does remember that he doesn't have to do anything quickly. That suits him just fine.

Doctor Garshowitz—Two weeks later

Roger's alone on the elevator, just back from lunch. The elevator stops on the third floor, and Dr. Garshowitz, the company doctor, gets on. Roger hasn't seen him since his last annual medical, before he was diagnosed.

"How're you doing, Roger?"

"Not so great. I'd like a word with you, if you have a minute."

Dr. Garshowitz nods. "Why don't we go to my office right now?"

Roger looks at his watch. So he'll be late for the meeting. "Okay."

At the office, Roger tells the doctor about what's happened, about his diagnosis. Then he asks the question he's been saving.

"I'd like to know why you didn't send me for a biopsy."

Dr. Garshowitz shrugs. "It was a judgement call. PSA readings can fluctuate over time. I thought we'd wait another year, and if it came back high I'd send you then. In hindsight, maybe I should have sent you sooner."

Roger nods. He figures it's the closest to an apology he's likely to get. "I've been thinking about what I should do next, but I'm not sure what would be best." It's not entirely the truth. Mostly he's been trying not to think about it. And he hasn't returned Dr. Martindale's phone calls. And Sarah's on his case big time. But what he remembers from the conversation with the doctor is that there's not a big hurry to decide.

Dr. Garshowitz is annoyed by Roger's nonchalant act, and he's privately upset with himself for not sending Roger for a biopsy sooner. He starts jabbing a finger in the air. "It sounds like you've known about this for weeks now, and you haven't taken any steps towards getting help. What's the matter with you? This is cancer, you know. It's serious stuff."

Roger can feel his anger rise in response. "It's not the end of the world. I've been told I can take my time making a decision."

"You've got to get on with the next step."

"So what's the next step?"

"You've got to go under the knife. That's the only sure way to deal with it. I want you to go and see a friend of mine, Dr. MacDonald. He can do your radical prostatectomy."

"Wait right there! I understood that there are other possibilities besides surgery."

"Not for a man your age. You need to get it out. So I'm going to set you up for an appointment. Okay?"

"Okay, but I'm still leaving my options open."

Then Dr. Garshowitz launches into a tirade about smoking, trying to convince Roger he should quit for the sake of his failing health. Roger listens for a few minutes, but that's all he can take.

"Is there any proof that smoking has anything to do with prostate cancer?"

"Well, there's no direct link that I know of, but ...."

Roger interrupts. "Then I don't want you to mention the word cigarette to me again. Clear?"

The doctor nods, not happy about it. "Okay, but I want you to see my urologist friend right away."

Doctor MacDonald—Two weeks later

Another waiting room. This time Sarah's with him. She says she doesn't trust him on his own, that he can't be relied on to deal with the things he needs to deal with. He can't understand what her problem is, but he's glad for the company. She has a big file of information piled on her lap, all downloaded from the Internet. As far as he's concerned, it's too much information. He's given up trying to read it, leaves it up to her. Besides, he figures it's the doctors' job to help make the decision.

A nurse comes to talk with them. She says that they should be sure not to interrupt the doctor when he talks with them, because he gets very annoyed. Roger raises his eyebrows. Sarah elbows him in the ribs. They both agree.

The nurse ushers them into Dr. MacDonald's office. Unsmiling, the doctor peers at them over bifocals. "Please have a seat. I'm going to explain some things to you now, and I'd ask you not to interrupt until I'm done."

He starts talking, and Roger is quickly lost. The doctor's using all these words he's unfamiliar with. He interrupts, asks a question. Dr. MacDonald looks at him severely. "Hold on a minute; wait until I'm finished."

Roger can't believe it, but doesn't see that he has a choice. The doctor continues. He draws graphs, makes pictures. Roger understands some of it, but is really glad that Sarah is taking notes as they go. The doctor explains the upsides and downsides for surgery, radiation treatment, and watchful waiting. When he finishes, he looks at Sarah's file of information, tells her to throw it away. Says that what he's provided is all the information they need, but that he'd be happy to arrange for them to talk with a radiation specialist if they want.

Sarah asks some questions, and the doctor answers them patiently. Roger isn't listening any more. He wants to go home. Dr. MacDonald seems to sense that he's lost his main audience.

"Why don't you go home and think about what I've said. Then come back and tell me what you've decided. If you want to have another opinion, call my nurse, and she'll arrange it."

"Thanks very much." Roger's out the door before Sarah can get to her feet.

Doctor MacDonald—Two weeks later

The doctor looks over his glasses at them. "So what have you decided?"

"I want you to do the operation." Roger's watching Sarah out of the corner of his eye. She's still annoyed at him for not going for another opinion. But it's his body, and he knows what he wants.

"Okay. Then let's schedule it."

"I want you to know that I have faith in your skills, that I'm impressed by your track record." Roger has checked Dr. MacDonald out thoroughly since their first meeting. His business experience has taught him that you hire somebody because they know how to do the job.

Dr. MacDonald doesn't respond, clearly not excited about being flattered about his work.

But Roger doesn't just want to flatter. "I'd prefer to have a friendly doctor who could make conversation and show a little human interest." No response, so he continues. "But if I have to choose I'd pick somebody with surgical skills over a great conversationalist." Roger waits to see if he'll get a response. The doctor is looking at him, not a muscle moving on his face, his hands shuffling papers on his desk.

Roger gives up on the hope of having rapport with his surgeon. Sarah's relieved that he does.

Doctor Chan—Four weeks later

Roger looks at his watch. Twenty after seven. Operation's set for 8 a.m. Suddenly, everything he's avoided thinking about for the past few weeks comes flooding in. What's going to happen? Will the surgery go all right? He's never had an operation before. He doesn't know what to expect. He wonders how he'll feel this time tomorrow. Then he wonders if he'll be around this time tomorrow.

A young man in a white coat enters.

"Hi, I'm Dr. Chan. I'm your anesthetist." He looks tired, which Roger figures can't be a good sign. "I just wanted to check to see if you wanted an epidural before we go into the operating room."

"What's that?"

"Oh, it's just a shot in the spine to help with the pain."

"They are putting me to sleep, aren't they?" Roger can feel his panic rising.

"Yes, yes. Don't worry. Some people just like a little extra help."

"I don't think so. It's bad enough you're going for my prostate. You're not going to get my spine too." Roger tries to make it into a joke.

Dr. Chan smiles wearily. "That's fine."

Roger sticks out his hand. "I want to shake your hand." The doctor complies.

"You're a very important man. I need you to do your job well. I don't want to wake up in the middle of this."

"Don't worry. Now I have to go. I'll see you in a few minutes."

Roger waits. He hates waiting. Finally, a nurse arrives. They walk together towards the surgery room.

"What, no limousine service for your patients?" He's trying to keep it light.

His mind turns to jails and executions, to hangings, to gas chambers. His knees feel weak.

The nurse seems to sense it.

"It's not that bad. You're in good hands here."

He wants to believe her. Wants to live a while longer.

Inside the operating room, he follows instructions and lies on the table. He's surprised at how narrow it is, hopes he won't fall off. He looks around the room but doesn't see Dr. MacDonald.

"Where's Dr. MacDonald?"

Dr. Chan answers. "He'll be here shortly." Then he starts wrapping up Roger's arm. He has a needle in his hand.

"I'd like you to start counting backwards from 100."

Roger breathes in, says a little prayer. Then he starts, "100, 99, 98...."

MEN'S HEALTH ATTITUDES AND PRACTICES

In recent years there has been a growing interest in men's health, fuelled by an increased awareness that many men are in trouble with health issues. For every age group, male mortality is higher than that of females. Life expectancy is lower for men. Men use primary health services, like family physicians, less than women do, and they are more likely to delay help-seeking when ill.[1] They are also more likely to adopt "risky" behaviors like drinking, smoking, violence, and fast driving and are less likely to engage in health-promoting activities.[2,3]

Poorer health outcomes for men can partly be traced to attitudes towards health and illness. In order to be the way that most men are taught they should be—i.e., independent, self-reliant, strong, robust, and tough—men are often willing to risk their health in unwise ways.[4]

Professional health care practices may also contribute to men's health problems. Research studies have shown that men typically receive significantly less physician time in their health visits than women do[5,6] *and receive fewer services.*[7] *Men are provided with fewer and briefer explanations in medical encounters and receive less advice from physicians about changing risk factors for disease.*[5,6] *While this is not always a problem, at least some of the time men's health problems may be overlooked because both men and their health professionals avoid discussing possible points of "weakness."*

REFERENCES

1. Kandrack, M., Grant, K. R., & Segall, A. (1991). Gender differences in health related behavior: Some unanswered questions. *Social Science and Medicine, 32*, 579-590.

2. Powell-Griner, E., Anderson, J. E., & Murphy, W. (1997). State- and sex-specific prevalence of selected characteristics ... behavioral risk factor surveillance system, 1994 and 1995. *Morbidity and Mortality Weekly Report, Centers for Disease Control, Surveillance Summaries, 46*, 1-31.

3. Shi, L. (1998). Sociodemographic characteristics and individual health behaviors. *Southern Medical Journal, 91*, 933-941.

4. Courtenay, W. H. (2000). Constructions of masculinity and their influence on men's well-being: A theory of gender and health. *Social Science and Medicine, 50*, 1385-1401.

5. Waitzkin, H. (1984). Doctor-patient communication: Clinical implications of social scientific research. *Journal of the American Medical Association, 252*, 2441-2446.

6. Weisman, C. S., & Teitelbaum, M. A. (1989). Women and health care communication. *Patient Education and Counseling, 13*, 183-199.

7. Verbrugge, L. M., & Steiner, R. P. (1985). Prescribing drugs to men and women. *Health Psychology, 4*, 79-98.

I'll Sail Away

*The speaker is a 64-year-old white man, treated
with radiation therapy nine months ago, currently
with no evidence of active disease. He is married
and has recently retired.*

I was born in a city on the east coast of England. We lived near the
docks. So for me, from the beginning, there were always ocean and
ships.

We were very poor.
My mother went out to work as a scrub lady.
She was very strict. She beat the hell out of us.
She had pressures.

It was an awful life. She had nothing in her life. I don't think she
ever went to a restaurant, never went on a vacation. It was always
scrape and scrounge, scrape and scrounge.
But still, she was very generous.

She was a terror. She was a spitfire.
I remember one night when the bombers were flying over. The people next door had their lights on in their house. So my mother went
out and yelled at them to turn out the lights. The lady next door
came flying out and started yelling back at my mother. They had a
fistfight right there on the street while the bombs were coming
down. They started beating each other with the lids of garbage cans.

I was killing myself laughing.

She started to work at city hall scrubbing halls when she was 56.
She was so good they kept her till she was 76. And she was still
going strong.

Nobody else understood her. They just thought she was a crabby old
bag, but she had a load to carry. They couldn't see it.
Only I could see it. I had great respect for her.

My father was totally different. He was very laid back. I guess
they'd call him cool today. Everybody loved him.
He was badly shot up in the First World War. So he couldn't work.
He never disciplined us, never hit us, nothing.
But he never gave us anything either, you know. Like at Christmas,
it was only my mother that gave to us. I sort of resented him. He
didn't carry his load. Even the discipline, she had to do it.
That was his job, a man's job.

I was very fiery.
I was in fights at school every day.
I was cock of the school, so I had to fight everybody.
It was a wild time.
Kids were real kids, not the pampered kind you find today.

Most of the friends I have today came from back then. Guys I
fought with on the streets.
I never backed down. That was part of it, never to back down. To
always go for it.
You get your nose bloodied, a black eye, whatever. It's just part of
the game.
For the people who live on the streets, it's the normal way of life.

When I was 14, the principal came into the classroom.
He said, "Get the hell out of here; you're finished."
That was the system. On your birthday, you were finished with

school. I was delighted. Ran all the way home.

One night, my mother and father were sitting there reading the paper
by the fire, and I said, "I'm running away to sea."
They said, "Oh, are you?"
I said, "Yeah." I had a handkerchief, and I had a toothbrush and a
little toy car, and those were my worldly possessions. So I said,
"Look, I'm off." Well, they just said, "Have a good time." That was
their attitude. Like not concerned, no reaction whatsoever.
So I walked out the door and took a streetcar down to the docks. I
crept past the police at the gate, got into the warehouse, and hid
behind a crate next to the gangway to the ship. When the guard went
to the toilet, I snuck on board the ship and got into the lifeboat. And
that's how it started.

It's not like my parents didn't care. It just wasn't a big thing like it
would be these days. The British army and navy were full of 14-year
olds.
I wasn't the only one.
There were lots of kids like me on the ships.

I was in the navy for three years and the army for five. I'm used to a
disciplined environment.
I was always confident in myself, my whole life. I didn't need a
crutch.
When I was in the army, I had to live in a hut with 30 men and eat
rotten food. Later on, there was a time I was completely broke and
had to live in my car. It didn't bother me.
I think adversity makes you stronger. I've always believed that, and
I think it's true.

I was always excellent in my job.
I had the fire in my guts.
When I went out to do something, I did it. Didn't matter how hard

or how long—I did it. Selling vacuum cleaners, I was the top salesman. And that's gotta be the hardest job in the world. But I did it.
I wasn't going to be beaten.

I was general manager for our company's Canadian division. All the
managers would meet in England twice a year. The top man there
took us to these private clubs in London. Very swishy places with all
these old fogies sitting around. And I'm getting introduced as the
Canadian manager. Everybody would shake my hand and look
impressed, and I'd think, you stupid buggers. You know, I'm a street
kid from the docks, and here you are associating with me as if I were
one of you. If you guys knew where I came from, you'd throw me
out.

I hate wimpy people. People who are timid and afraid and who don't
stand up for themselves. They get pushed around and just accept it.
I hate people like that.
I'm a guy that's pretty tough and strong and successful.

I had a heart attack a few years ago, and then I had a stroke. And
then I got diagnosed with prostate cancer.
I decided on the radiation therapy.
One of the side effects of the treatment was impotence.
I'm pretty strong-minded, and I can switch my thoughts. If I get
negatives I start to switch to something positive.

I've stopped going to the prostate cancer support group. I find that
there are negative people there. You hear some of these case histo-
ries that don't work out. That's not a very positive thing. So once I
got all the information I needed, I stopped listening to anybody else.

I think that you can continue on fighting this disease as long as you
look for new directions and try new things. And there's lots of them
coming up every day.

Since I've been diagnosed with prostate cancer, I've been very, very
strong. I just carried on with life.
I took a lot of vitamins and stuff.
I felt good, and I just wrote the prostate cancer off.
I think it's down to my natural optimism. I'm very strong in my
mind; I can make my mind go in whichever direction I want it to go.
Ten people can have prostate cancer, and it can affect them in ten
different ways. And some of it's related to the person himself.
I think mind over matter is a major factor.
I've applied mind over matter a lot.

Once this is all done with, I'm going to get a job on a cruise ship
and go back to sea. For maybe six months or a year.
It's sort of a last chance. I've always wanted to do it.
My wife's not interested. She has the grandchildren, and she concen-
trates on them. That's her life. Those are her priorities.
I have mine.
I don't think I'll miss my family too much.
I've always been the kind of guy who fits into an environment and
becomes part of it. Wherever I am, that's where I am. I don't think
of other places and other things. It was like that in the army too.
I never get homesick.
It's not like I'm trying to get away from my wife.
I'm just going towards what I want.

I don't fear it.
I know I've probably got no more than five to ten years.
My ambition was always to die at 96, shot by a jealous husband.
So, I may not make it to 96.

My whole life I've been an individual.
I'll do my thing, and you do yours.
I won't tell you what to do.
Don't tell me what to do.

ABOUT MASCULINITY

Masculinity has traditionally been defined in western cultures by characteristics such as competitiveness, aggression, independence, stoicism, and rationalism.[1] Often it has been assumed that men are biologically or socially programmed to be this way, that we really have little choice in the matter—or that if men do exercise other options it's merely a failure in achieving "real" masculinity. But this belief about how men have to be is not universally accepted. Recent writing in the social sciences argues for many more possibilities for men and their expressions of masculinity. It emphasizes the active way that men participate in shaping or "performing" masculinity and also reveals how masculinity is fluctuating and fluid rather than fixed and permanent.[2]

If men have options about how to be masculine and can make real choices other than the traditional, then this is relevant to their health. Traditional ways of being "masculine," while arguably bringing advantages to some life domains (such as business), tend to undermine possibilities for health and limit men's experiences related to illness. Real men, after all, are supposed to be unconcerned about health matters. Real men don't fuss about their bodies.[3] Real men don't need help. Men who identify most strongly with these traditional masculine values have been shown to engage in poorer health behaviors and to take greater health risks than other men with less traditional values.[4] Men's ability to deal with prostate cancer may partly depend upon how willing they are to reconsider masculinity and make room for new experiences and changed personal capacities.

References

1. Cheng, C. (1999). Marginalized masculinities and hegemonic masculinity: An introduction. *The Journal of Men's Studies, 7*, 295-315.

2. Connell, R.W. (1995). *Masculinities*. Berkeley: University of California Press.

3. Watson, J. M. (2002). *Male bodies: Health, culture and identity.* Philadelphia: Open University Press.

4. Courtenay, W. H. (2000). Constructions of masculinity and their influence on men's well-being. *A theory of gender and health. Social Science & Medicine, 50*, 1385-1401.

Maurice Runs a Meeting

Maurice is a 59-year-old white man who had a radical prostatectomy three years ago and is currently disease-free. He's married, recently retired, and a leader at the prostate cancer support group.

Maurice wipes around his mouth and then drops the tissue into the bowl, flushes for the second time. He hasn't heard anyone come in, but still looks around when he opens the cubicle door. He stands in front of the mirror, rinsing with the mouthwash he always brings. He brushes his thick gray hair.

"Thank God that's over with." He says it out loud.

Maurice is annoyed that it still happens every time. The guys in the group don't believe him when he tells them how nervous he gets about leading a meeting. Frank even told him his public speaking style was smooth as silk, which Maurice has to admit made him feel pretty good. It's always been this way, his fooling people into thinking he's on top of things. All those years as a manager, and nobody ever knowing about his struggles. It was part of the job to give the appearance of being in control. Bess calls it being a good bullshitter, and she's right about that.

He makes his way downstairs and into the hall. There are about 20 men so far and a few women. He greets the ones he knows by name. It's something he learned as a manager, that if you remember people's names they're more likely to forgive you your mistakes. He counts the wooden chairs set out in rows facing the front, making sure there will be enough. There were 200 at the last meeting, 180 the time before that. Somebody, probably Mavis, has the coffee urn set up and the red light is already on. John is setting out books and pamphlets on a table, waves a hand in Maurice's direction. Maurice shouts across the room at him.

"Everything you never wanted to know about prostate cancer, eh?" John shakes his head from side to side, confirming Maurice's bad attitude. Maurice has read a few of the books, or at least started a few of them. One of these days he will get around to doing more serious reading. Right. And maybe he'll give up beer and lose weight, too. Right.

A stout man in his mid-40s has made an entrance to the hall. Given that he's the only guy here under 55, and wearing an ill-fitting sport jacket and tie, Maurice figures it must be Dr. Harrington. He decides to check.

"Dr. Harrington?" A nod for confirmation.

"I'm Maurice Gardeaux. We spoke on the phone."

"Ah, yes. Pleased to meet you. I've got my slides here. Will we be starting soon?"

Doctors, they're always in a hurry. Maurice wonders, not for the first time, if manic people choose medicine, or if they only become manic afterwards.

"We'll start at 5 after 7 if that's all right with you. I'll welcome people and make a few announcements, and then I'll introduce you. Do you want to take some questions after your talk? The guys usually like that."

"That will be fine," the doctor says, looking anything but thrilled. "But I won't give medical advice on individual cases."

"Of course not." Heaven forbid.

Maurice fits the slide carousel into the machine, checks the microphone attached to the lectern, searches for his notes in his jacket pocket. He's still feeling nervous, but not as much as he was. He sits in the front row, watching people trickle in, the room slowly filling up with old men. He likes looking at them. It makes him feel kind of sentimental inside. They're like crusty old warriors, he muses, survivors of life's countless battles, fighting another one now.

He surprised himself during that research interview the other day with how passionate he sounded about the group, about the possibilities for men helping men. Thinking about it now, he tries to remember exactly what he said. Something about how this is his moment, his time, and the group is the place where he's making his mark. Who'd have ever thought he'd get that worked up about a bunch of old farts. A few years ago he would have run the other way.

At exactly four minutes after seven, Maurice moves to the lectern, reads from the notes he carefully prepared two nights ago. He explains the schedule for the evening, points out the coffee and books for those who might have missed them, gives a plug for the speakers for the next few meetings, and announces that there's a new study about the effects of Vitamin E and selenium on prostate cancer and that people can pick up a flyer on the table over there. Then he reads the introduction that the doctor's secretary faxed him yesterday. Dr. Harrington is a radiation oncologist with an impressive array of credentials. He'll be talking about conformal radiotherapy, new advances, and future possibilities. Please, everyone, join him in welcoming Dr. Harrington.

Back in his seat, Maurice is instantly more relaxed. He intends to listen, even leans forward to concentrate. But there are too many slides with too many graphs and numbers. And to be honest, he's not really interested in any of the fancy new radiotherapy techniques. He made another choice a long time ago, went for the surgery. That's what Bess wanted, insisted that he take the best chance for cure and to hell with sex. He appreciated her point, thankful that she wanted him alive no matter what the cost.

Maurice finds himself remembering the first time he came to the group. He was nervous then, too, nervous about the very idea of men's groups, about the possibility they might breed homosexuality. He knew the fear was probably stupid, but God knows he didn't want anything to do with that kind of nonsense. He'd also been worried about other men knowing about his situation, the constant flooding, and how humiliated he felt by it all. For other men to know about his weakness went against everything he'd learned growing up, everything that had been required to survive in his work. Men in the company knew that you couldn't let other guys know too much about you. Sooner or later they'd use it against you, undermine your ability to compete.

He probably never would have taken the step of coming to that first meeting if Fred and Norman hadn't visited him while he was still in hospital. He appreciated their taking the time, and they seemed like normal kinds of guys. He told them he would come to the group once he was up to it, but it took him four months to follow through. By that time Bess was on his case, telling him in her usual sweet way to get his head out of his ass and do something to help himself. God, he loves that woman.

Despite his hesitations, the group turned out to be a lifesaver. Right off the top he got a few tips that helped with his incontinence. But the really big thing for Maurice was the feeling that he wasn't alone, that other guys were in the same boat. It shouldn't have been such a revelation, but it was.

Bess had been stunned by his sudden enthusiasm for the group. After his second meeting, he was smoking and drinking beer in the kitchen and feeling pretty good and got almost eloquent about it.

"It's as if all those men at the meeting are naked, made equal by prostate cancer. It doesn't matter whether you're a doctor or a production guy or an unemployed guy. You're still sitting there like the rest, with short little penises that don't work properly. Nobody's saying, 'my prostate's bigger than yours.' There's just nothing to be competitive about. All that stuff about how men usually are with men just seems to disappear."

Bess had gotten quiet after his little speech, and later they'd had a bit of a cuddle. He'd like to be able to come up with another eloquent speech after the meeting tonight.

Dr. Harrington is behaving as if he's coming to the end of his talk, predicting that the universal "we" will continue to improve treatments in the coming years. Well, that would be nice, thinks Maurice, but what about a cure or, even better, preventing the blasted disease? The last graph departs from the screen at the front of the room, leaving an empty square of white light. The doctor invites response from his numbed audience. It's the usual hodge-podge of questions, none of them directly relevant to the talk they've just been subjected to. Men taking the golden opportunity to try one more time to get answers for the things they haven't been able to get information about, things they haven't been able to understand even when they did get the information.

What is an abnormal PSA level? The doctor says it all depends on age.

Does the doctor recommend the alternative treatment PC-SPES? He doesn't, points out that it has been withdrawn from the market because of possible contamination.

Are there dietary changes the doctor recommends? He doesn't say, says there needs to be more research.

Does the doctor think radiation is better than surgery? He equivocates.

Maurice stands to thank Dr. Harrington for his stimulating presentation. The men join him in warm applause, in acknowledging the importance of doctors coming to the meetings. It's a demonstration of interest and commitment. And they bring with them the information that all these guys are desperate for. That's what makes these meetings so successful, Maurice muses, the possibility of the disease becoming comprehensible, the possibility of finding that right piece of information that will make it all go away. Maurice knows that information is critical for the guys, and for him too, but he still sometimes wishes more attention were paid to other stuff.

As soon as the break is official, the men all make for the wash-room like stampeding buffalo. Maurice stays back to get the doctor his slides, thanks him again for coming. He walks the doctor to the door and is about to step out to have a smoke when he spies Fred seated at the back of the room. Fred's one of the guys who visited him that first time in hospital, and it's been a few months since he's been to a meeting. To Maurice, he looks frail and somehow smaller. He follows his impulse and crosses the room in Fred's direction.

"Hi, Fred. It's really good to see you." Fred stands slowly to shake hands, wincing almost imperceptibly, his smile looking strained.

"Hello yourself, Maurice. I didn't know you were such an accomplished public speaker."

"You know how it is. They couldn't find anybody else, so I got conscripted."

"Well, they made a good choice. Anyway, I've been hearing that you retired from your job. How are you finding the life of leisure?"

"Best decision I ever made. Should have done it long ago." This is Maurice's standard line, and he feels a bit sheepish offering it up to Fred. So he quickly moves to change the focus.

"How about you, Fred? How have you been?"

Fred shrugs, loses his smile, looks down at the floor. Maurice wonders if his question is intrusive.

"The past few months have been a bit tough for me and Liz. The hormones aren't working the way they were." He looks up at Maurice, his face struggling to reconfigure itself into the smile.

"But it could be worse. And we're off to Ottawa in a couple of weeks for my grandson's wedding. It'll take more than a little pain in my bones to keep me away from that."

Maurice tries to keep his voice sounding cheerful.

"Sounds like fun. That's the grandson you're so fond of, is it?"

Fred nods.

"I hope you and Liz have a great time. But I am sorry to hear you haven't been feeling well." There's a brief silence while Maurice fights with himself. He wants to respect Fred's right to privacy, his right to suffer alone, but he also wants to reach out somehow, without making it look like he thinks Fred needs help.

"Would you mind if I dropped around some afternoon for coffee? I could use a bit of company now that I have more time on my hands."

Fred looks pleased. "I'd like that, Maurice. Maybe I can give you a few pointers on being retired. Like how to avoid your wife murdering you for being underfoot all the time."

Maurice laughs. "Maybe I'd better drop by soon. That sounds like something I need to learn." He glances at his watch. "I guess I'd better get the small groups going. Let's be in touch."

As he walks away from Fred, Maurice feels bad. Bad because he didn't get out for a smoke and he really needed one. Bad because Fred's disease is obviously getting worse. Bad because he thinks he owes it to Fred to be more honest about his own situation. Truth is, he's not sure at all that he made the right decision by retiring from work. But he puts on a show of knowing, giving himself some space to sort it out privately. That's the way he did it with the prostate cancer too, not letting people know he was reeling from the news. In the weeks after his diagnosis, he joked about it, pretended to treat it lightly. He even fooled himself to some degree, thought he was doing just fine, until one of his friends lambasted him for not taking things seriously enough. That sobered him up, so to speak.

It's part of a larger question that he's been musing about: whether he's being the right kind of man. Partly he thinks men should be straightforward, willing to lay things on the line. And he can do that sometimes, especially here at the meeting, and more and more with his close friends, too. But mostly, he'd rather that other people don't know about his handicap. Is he being a coward? Or is it better to keep some things to yourself? God knows, John Wayne wouldn't have told everyone that he had to wear pads and couldn't get stiff.

There are six guys in Maurice's group, chairs moved into a circle. It turns out that Fred is one of them, and he gives Maurice a wink. Maurice is the facilitator for the group, having once taken a day-long training session offered by the cancer society. He's forgotten most of the training now because it was just stuff about how to get guys to say something, making sure everybody gets a chance to talk. Not exactly rocket science.

Maurice asks everybody to introduce himself, say a few words about his situation. Two of the guys, Jerry and Max, are recently diagnosed and, from the looks on their faces, scared as hell. The rest of them make sympathetic noises, having all been in that place of trying to figure out up from down. Another guy, Nick, is near the end of his radiation treatment and wants to know if other guys had trouble with diarrhea and what brand of diapers they use. Then there's

Wally, whom Maurice knows from other group discussions. Wally is what you could call a challenge for group facilitators because he knows everything and wants to convince other guys of what he knows. He was diagnosed a couple of years ago and has yet to have any conventional treatment. A "watchful waiter," he's been monitoring his PSA test results and doing every kind of alternative treatment under the sun. The last time Wally was in Maurice's group, he tried to convert the other guys to a macrobiotic diet. Maurice finally told him to back off, told him that every man had the right to make his own choices and not feel judged. Then he tried to turn it into a joke, saying he happened to be big on hot dogs and beer, and he thought that must be an anti-cancer diet because he put lots of ketchup on the hot dogs, and doesn't Wally know that research shows that tomatoes are good for preventing prostate cancer.

After the introductions, the conversation focuses on Jerry and Max and their attempts to decide about treatment. Maurice can sense how they all want to help these guys. Everybody trots out his treatment story. When it's Maurice's turn, he speaks bluntly.

"I was scared to death of the surgery. I mean, nobody knew I was, but I still was. And I'm not real good about pain, so I made the docs swear that they'd make sure I had lots of medication."

Jerry and Max both look kind of startled with Maurice's revelations. Fred is smiling in his direction, having heard it before.

"I was pretty worried about everything. And to be honest I had a few tears about it. I know that men aren't supposed to cry, but sometimes it's just the natural thing. If either of you guys ever feels the need to cry while you're going through this stuff, don't you worry about it. Lots of men have been there before you."

Their faces are blank, not giving any indication that they know what Maurice is talking about, that they might be the kind of guys who would ever need such advice. Maurice takes a deep breath. He decided some time back that he wanted to say these kinds of things, so that other men wouldn't feel as alone with their struggles as he had. But it still scares him to do it. Like now, feeling like he's made himself too vulnerable, that maybe they see him as a wimp. He should behave more like the other group leaders and stick to the straight information. Talking about feelings just makes everybody uncomfortable. God knows he's uncomfortable. And he really needs a smoke.

Max breaks the short silence following Maurice's speech, says he wants to ask about impotence. His doctor has told him not to worry too much about it because there are things that can be done to help even if he turns out to be impotent and, besides, with nerve-sparing surgery there's a good chance there won't be a problem. Fred makes eye contact with Maurice and gives a little shrug. These poor suckers don't have a clue what they're in for. Maurice shrugs his agreement.

Nick takes the standard approach, saying how the most important thing is to do whatever it takes to stay alive. Everybody nods. Hard to disagree with that. Fred leans forward, elbow resting on a thin leg, opens his mouth to speak.

"I thought by choosing radiation, I'd get away without the side effects, but it didn't turn out that way. Back when I was diagnosed, we didn't have Viagra. But we did try the vacuum pump. What a waste of money that was. We never could figure out how to use the blasted thing."

Jerry chuckles nervously, not sure if this should be funny or not.

"Next we tried the injections. It took five or six times before we got the dosage right." Fred grimaces. "Anyway, we finally got it working and had a couple of years doing that. But then I started these bloody hormones. Now, the Playmate-of-the-Month could walk in here without a stitch on, and I'd just yawn."

Maurice laughs with Fred, but finds the story hard to hear. The thought of losing his sex drive is almost as scary as the thought of the cancer coming back. He can't imagine not being able to get worked up about Bess. Sometimes she'll just be cooking dinner, wearing some old thing, and he'll be panting like a dog he gets so turned on. And just yesterday at the burger joint, making eyes at the curvy little brunette behind the counter. Imagining what it would be like to sneak off for a cuddle. Not that he would. He has his rules about that kind of thing. And, besides, Bess would kill him. But he sure likes to think about doing it, likes to push the flirting right up to the edge.

The conversation has momentarily stalled. Maurice seizes the moment.

"The thing is, guys, that even if you do end up impotent and even if the Viagra or whatever else doesn't work, it doesn't have to mean the end of your sex life. It just calls for more creativity."

They're all looking at him expectedly, waiting for more details. But Maurice decides to leave it at that. Last meeting he offended a couple of those religious types when he told them that as long as you've got ten fingers and a tongue sex can still be alive and well. Bess hooted when he told her about that, couldn't believe that he would come out with such a thing in public. But she did agree it was true, did tell him yet again that he's probably a better lover now than before the operation. And that's really going some. Sometimes he thinks Bess is an even bigger bullshitter than he is. And that's really going some.

Maurice remembers what else he wants to say.

"I'm not going to say it's easy to be impotent, but there are lots of guys in this room who are dealing with it pretty well. Have you guys talked to your wives about this?"

Max nods, but Jerry flinches, looking like this is the last thing he wants to talk about. Maurice feels the familiar doubt, the worry that he's pushed too hard. What right does he have to intrude like this?

Jerry rubs his hands through thinning blond hair. "I wouldn't know what to say. It just seems so unfair that she might have to go without sex because of what happens to me."

Fred jumps in ahead of Maurice. "Find a quiet moment and take her aside and tell her about how you feel. Wives are usually pretty understanding about these kinds of things."

"Yeah," says Maurice, "they're not as obsessed with our erections as we like to think. And she's not going to think you're not a man if you can't perform like a teenager any more."

Maurice has seen it again and again over the past few years, how women seem to adapt fairly easily to the loss of sex. But men don't do nearly as well. God knows Bess seems to be doing better than he is. But maybe she just doesn't talk about it, like he doesn't talk to her about his sense of feeling handicapped, about how he sometimes can't get the thought out of his head that he's not a real man any more. Even though he knows better. He knows that being a man is mostly about other stuff like taking a stand when it's necessary, looking out for the people you care about, but it still creeps in. Sometimes he wonders if he'll ever stop feeling like a cripple.

Maurice looks at his watch, sees there are only five minutes left. He's halfway out of his chair, but that's when Wally starts to talk, a shaky quality to his voice that Maurice hasn't heard before. Wally avoids making eye contact.

"I had my PSA done last week, and it's gone up, quite a lot. So I've made an appointment to go and see the urologist. I guess my time of watching and waiting is over. I really thought the macrobiotic diet would cure me."

Maurice sinks back onto the chair. Sadness washes over him.

"I'm sorry to hear that, Wally. Maybe your diet slowed the cancer down, bought you some extra time. You never know."

Wally gives Maurice a wan smile. And then Nick asks Wally about what treatment he's going to have. Maurice excuses himself and walks to the front of the hall, turns on the microphone. He announces that it's time to wrap things up. He reminds everyone about the date of the next meeting, encourages them to show up.

Usually Maurice stands around and visits at the end of a meeting, but tonight he's absolutely desperate for that smoke. He lights up as soon as he's out of the front door. Such moments make life worth living.

A few of the guys pass him on the way to the parking light, exchange "good nights." Then suddenly Max is standing in front of him.

"Maurice, I wanted to thank you for your comments in the

group. When I came here tonight, I was feeling pretty sorry for myself. Now I realize I'm not the only catfish in the lake. And, thanks to you, I'm not so worried about the couple of times I broke down at work. I thought maybe I was having a nervous breakdown or something."

"It's hard to keep this bloody disease from getting to you once in awhile." Maurice is beaming, feeling even better than when he lit the cigarette. He offers his hand to Max. They shake and say good-night. Alone again, Maurice shakes his head in wonder. What a great thing this group is! And showing weakness to other guys seems to pay off. What a blast it is to help!

He thinks of Bess, how he wants to tell her all about what Max said. But maybe he'll first stop and grab a quick pint on the way home. A pint would definitely go really well about now. Bess will give him hell, but she'll understand, will be waiting for him when he gets in. God, he loves that woman.

MEN HELPING MEN?

Research has shown that most men disclose little about their everyday struggles to other men.[1] Men's chronic competitiveness in relationships usually keeps them from revealing their losses of control and their points of vulnerability.[2] This can be even more pronounced in the situation of illness, where men can often feel somehow less than other men. Most men in our studies expressed hesitations about whether, and how much, they wanted other men to know about their prostate cancer experiences.

Despite the concerns that men often hold about other men, prostate cancer support groups have flourished in North America. These groups first appeared in the early 1990s and have now spread all over the U.S. and Canada. In the U.S., the two main organizations are Us Too and Man to Man.³ In Canada, most local groups belong to an umbrella organization, the Canadian Prostate Cancer Network.⁴ The main purpose of these groups is to provide men better access to information about prostate cancer and its treatment. Most groups sponsor talks by medical experts and also provide the opportunity for men with prostate cancer to debate issues through small group discussions. Spouses are often integrally involved with the groups. In some groups wives meet separately from their husbands while in other groups men and women participate together. Members report high satisfaction with groups.⁵

In interviews we conducted with leaders of prostate cancer groups, men clearly identified access to information as the key issue facing patients.⁶ They (unlike the women we interviewed in breast cancer groups) did not consider emotional support or intimate sharing to be a main focus for the groups, although most were pleasantly surprised about the connections they made with other men.

Despite men's downplaying of the importance of support and friendship within prostate cancer groups, these groups represent a challenge to men's usual ways of dealing with illness. Men do seem able to help each other in important ways.

REFERENCES

1. Notarius, C., & Johnson, J. (1982). Emotional expression in husbands and wives. *Journal of Marriage and Family, 44,* 483-489.

2. Naifeh, S., & Smith, G. (1984). *Why can't men open up? Overcoming men's fear of intimacy.* New York: Clarkson N. Potter.

3. Us Too International's mailing address is: 930 North York Road, Suite 50, Hinsdale, IL 60521-2993. (Website: www.ustoo.com). Man to Man's address is: American Cancer Society, 1599 Clifton Road,

N.E., Atlanta, GA 30329-4251. (Website: www.cancer.org/m2m.htm/).

4. Canadian Prostate Cancer Website is: www.cpcn.org.

5. Coreil, J., & Behal, R. (1999). Man to Man prostate cancer support groups. *Cancer Practice, 7*, 122-129.

6. Gray, R. E., Fitch, M., Davis, C., & Phillips, C. (1997). Interviews with men with prostate cancer about their self-help group experience. *Journal of Palliative Care, 13*, 15-21.

Carl Retreats to the Den

Carl is a 70-year-old black man, in the process of deciding on radiation therapy for his recently diagnosed prostate cancer. He is married and has retired from a warehouse job.

Monday

"I'm going into the den for a while." Carl's voice is deep and strong for such a small man, filling the apartment. She looks up from the kitchen sink, startled. Probably, he thinks, wondering why he announced it as if it were unusual. He's not sure why. After all, he's done the same thing day in and day out for years, since the kids were babies and even before. Carl folds the newspaper, adds it to the recycling pile, pushes his chair back from the table, grabs his cane. She has dried her hands and is standing beside him, dark fingers light on his arm, ready to help.

"I'm not an invalid yet." The fingers pull away. He senses her watching him as he makes his way slowly across the kitchen, knows he should turn and say something civil. But the resentment is too strong right now, resentment of her but not just her. She watches him go, knowing it will do no good to reach out, wishing things were less difficult.

He switches on the lamp, sinks into the cushioned chair. Papers covered with his tiny script, legible only to him, are scattered across the wooden desk. He knows there's no point in trying to work on the manuscript tonight. Nor does he feel inclined to open the book about

Mahatma Gandhi, no matter that he was enjoying it so much last night, remembering the passion he'd had as a younger man, the first time he'd read it. He closes his eyes, decides to pray, reaching out to God.

But his mind doesn't go to God. Instead, it goes back to the doctor's office. He'd known it couldn't be good news when he was asked to come in after the biopsy. She'd known too, had insisted on coming with him. The doctor, not a bad guy but not much of a conversationalist, got right to the point. Prostate cancer. Carl was surprised at the strength of the tremor that rushed through him. The doctor carried on talking, but Carl didn't take much of it in. Some stuff about the different treatments he could have, the pros and cons of each. She had asked questions, Carl impatient with her and just wanting to get out of the office and go home. For some reason, he'd started thinking about his old mom and how she was at the end, wasted away and moaning in pain for months. No way he wanted to go through that, put the family through that. Thinking about it, he felt like he might start crying right there in front of the doctor, totally humiliate himself.

Even now he doesn't get why he's had such a strong reaction to having cancer. After all his study of religion, he'd thought he would be ready to accept the natural course of things. It's embarrassing, this unexpected weakness, this desire of an old man to live forever.

He turns his mind deliberately towards the prospect of death, determined to confront the fear. An image from the past whirls into view. His elder brother, Jake, later killed in the war, is holding him out over the end of the pier, insistent that Carl learn to swim. Even now, sitting in his old man's chair, he feels the terror of flying through the air, bony arms and legs flailing vainly in the attempt to avoid the waiting lake. And the going up and going down and desperate gulping for air, but getting only water. And the surprising sweet peace invading his tiring body, so that it was almost disappointing when Jake's right arm dragged him spluttering to shore.

Somehow the memory has made it easier to pray. Carl thanks God for bringing him a bit of peace about his cancer, tells God to come and get him whenever it's time. He sits quietly, trying to sense the presence of God; at moments is sure he can feel Him. After a while, he reaches over to turn the lamp off. She's already asleep when he gets to bed.

Tuesday

When the time arrives, he doesn't make an announcement. He just folds the paper and heads in the direction of the den.

She doesn't look up from the sink, knows his rhythms like her own heartbeat. She's aware of how quiet he's been today, so unlike him. Usually he has something to say about everything. She realizes she's worried about him. It's not a big surprise to be worried. It's what women do, she thinks, what she was brought up to do. But she hadn't been ready to feel this way about him, has been startled by the flickers of hope. Maybe her love has just been in hiding, not gone like she'd thought. She's been teetering on the edge of telling him how she's feeling. But she's afraid, not wanting to be pulled back into his orbit, not wanting the sexual expectations to start all over again. Maybe it's best to leave things alone.

Carl is oblivious to her, anxious to finish the work he started in the morning. Sorting the books into piles on the floor of the den, slipping pieces of paper inside the covers, each paper with a name scrawled on it. Some, not many, have the name of one his children: Janet, Don, Marilyn. Mostly, though, they aren't interested in history or philosophy or religion, don't understand his passion for ideas. They resented the time he was away from the family at evening classes. But it had been that way for him since he was a boy and spent his spare time in the school library. He'd ignored the teacher's suggestion to concentrate on woodworking, resented the implication that it was a practical vocation for a poor, skinny black kid. Back then, he'd been certain his mother's labor scrubbing white women's kitchens so that her children could be educated wouldn't go to waste.

Most of the slips in the books show the names of younger men he's mentored, men from the community who appreciate what he understands. There is only the one slip with her name on it, inserted into a compilation of love poems that he bought for her many years ago, between Don and Janet. She'd stopped him from reading them out loud, too embarrassing, she'd said—indecent, too. Maybe she'd feel differently about them when he was gone. Maybe she'd feel differently about him, too.

Carl sighs, sinks lower in the chair, rubs his forehead with his middle finger. Just like his father had done, finally home from the sea, dry-eyed after the funeral of his wife, stroking his forehead over and over.

Wednesday

He is late getting to the den on account of the kids. It's hardly right to think about them as kids anymore, with all of them over 45, but he still does. It was awkward at first, them being worried about him but having trouble saying much about it. Carl wonders if it's his fault that they're such poor communicators.

They sat at the dining room table and drank tea and ate the strawberry tarts she'd made in the afternoon. Marilyn finally asked how he was doing and he said he was fine, nothing to worry about. Don wanted to know what treatment he was going to have, and it was obvious from the look on his face he wasn't happy that Carl hadn't decided yet. Predictably it was Don who continued to barge ahead and ask the questions that they were all thinking about: had a will been made, and would his mom be well taken care of, and what about other arrangements? Carl didn't mind being asked, was glad for the chance to show how well he'd prepared. After he laid it all out, the kids seemed relieved, and pretty soon they were talking about gardening, and then the Blue Jays, and then their kids. But Carl could tell that cancer was still there in the room. Eyes sought him out, then darted away. Janet, who had never helped in the kitchen without being asked, brought him the platter of tarts with a smile. And nobody made a snide comment when he took a third.

Tonight he's ready to read more about Gandhi. It's the chapter about the first long fast. Carl marvels at the man's courage, his readiness to embrace death in the service of peace. But he's still relieved when he gets to the point where the authorities make their concessions and Gandhi breaks the fast, takes some food. Carl finds himself in tears.

He closes the book, muses about why he's so moved, the resonance with his own situation. Now that he's laid out the plans for after his death, he feels released, pretty much ready to go. But he also feels a renewed surge of energy, a desire to squeeze out a few more good years. He thinks about Jeremy, who's been coming by weekly to talk with him about the history of black spirituality. Their last discussion was about the Haitian slave who broke the back of the French army during the early colonial period, about what it takes to be a leader when your people are oppressed. He wants more meetings with Jeremy. And he wants to finish that blasted manuscript he's been working on for 20 years.

Praying, he offers it up to God. Says he's ready to go whenever, but that he'd prefer an extension if that happened to fit in with God's will. He's smiling when he turns off the light.

Thursday

He's late again and thinks about going straight to bed but decides to spend a few minutes in the den first. It's because she talked him into going to the prostate support group meeting, trying anything to get him to make a decision about treatment. The speaker at the meeting, a specialist in radiation therapy, was pretty hard to follow. Too many slides with graphs on them, too many details. But he still learned a few things. Like how sexual problems seemed not to be as likely after radiation as after surgery. And that there's a new program for seed implant radiation treatment at a local hospital.

He wasn't surprised that there was only one other guy there from his community. But he was surprised at how welcoming all the white guys were. It reinforced what he likes to believe, that there is nobility within every person, and that to tap into that is to tap into our shared humanity, beyond skin color. It was so obvious sitting in the meeting that everyone was in the same boat. We all feel love, we all feel pain, we all feel rejection. And it was somehow reassuring to see all those other men, some of them years after treatment, still walking, talking, and smiling. He was glad she'd talked him into going.

Friday

Carl bangs the paper on the table, feeling the heat rise in his face.

"I can't believe this racist rag. You'd think in a so-called civilized country there'd be some sensitivity about these things. Bloody police chief, refusing to meet with leaders of the community, making out that they're just troublemakers. When you keep pushing people down, it's no wonder they start to stir up trouble. I want to cancel our subscription today!"

She turns towards him, away from the nuts she's chopping, eyebrows raised, a half-smile on her lips. This is more like the hot air balloon she's lived with so long, her man of principle, of noble ideals and outrage. He infuriates her in so many ways, but she admires his passion for justice. "And how many times would that make it for canceling the paper?"

"Don't you go making fun of me, woman." But he can't squelch a chuckle, seeing himself for just a moment through her eyes. Still, he doesn't want her thinking she's right.

"Look here, this section on world news. There's hardly anything about the slaughter in Rwanda, nothing at all about the drought in Ethiopia. No, ma'am, what we have is a big article about white landowners losing their ranches. As if three generations of exploiting the black man gives them the right to call Africa home. My God, there's more coverage for English cows than for Africans with AIDS."

She rolls her eyes and shrugs, turns back to the nuts. She knows he's right, of course, but she's heard it all a hundred times before. Carl slams the paper down again, leaves it on the table. She can bloody well put it in the recycling pile herself.

"I'm going to the den now!" He makes it clear he's had enough of her apathy. That's the whole trouble with the black community these days, too willing to let things go by. He comes just short of slamming the door.

He can't get comfortable in his chair, still seething inside. It's a familiar feeling. There was a time he was almost always like this, consumed with anger. Like when he worked on the trains. He finally knew he had to quit or hurt somebody, knew it when that last jowly guy in a suit called him boy and tossed a quarter in his direction, wanting Carl to get him a drink. He still marvels that he stopped himself from killing that guy. He's glad that he was smart enough to transfer to a warehouse and stay there. Maybe if things had been different he could have been a professor or a judge, made his mark as a black man in the world. But the war had come along and then the kids and … it hadn't turned out like he'd hoped, but he'd done all right. It would just have to do. Lots of poor skinny black boys have done worse in this hateful society.

He's thinking about the prostate group meeting last night, about how he'd been feeling so optimistic. Do men have to be sick or on the brink of death before they wake up to their common humanity? God, what a mess this world is.

Saturday

He's part way through an article about a judge accused of making racist comments, thinking about whether they were really racist, when he notices that she's looking at him. It's actually more like glaring, arms crossed and leaning against the stove. Just like she used to do when one of the kids screwed up. He tries to ignore her, to carry on reading. But she crosses to the table and sits directly opposite. Hard to ignore that. He looks up, ready for the worst.

"So have you made a decision about getting treatment for your cancer?" Her tone is soft, level, determined. She's thinking she's had enough. No more mucking about, mister. He doesn't even try to stall.

"I'm thinking I'll go for the radiation."

She raises her eyebrows, not pleased. He knows she thinks the evil should come out. But he still decides to try and convince her.

"They recommend radiation for most men my age. Surgery is usually for the younger ones. The doctor at the group meeting said radiation was about as effective as surgery."

She's listening, not convinced but considering.

"I'd rather not go back on the operating table if I can help it."

She nods, remembering the back surgery he had 15 years ago. How he was laid up for months and was such a pain to deal with. And his back wasn't even any better.

"So that's it, then? You're sure?" She's speaking to her lap.

"I'll talk to the doctor about it once more when we go back, but I'm pretty sure." He pauses, takes a deep breath. "The other thing is that with the radiation there's less chance of being impotent."

Her head snaps up, her eyes make fiery contact. But then she looks away. She's thinking about the last five years, about her decision to stop having sex. About her desire to be left alone, finally allowed some peace.

Suddenly, though, she wants him to hold her, like he used to do when she was upset. She almost moves to stroke his hand, almost says that she understands how he must feel. But the moment goes by, and she is silent, still unmoving. Then she gets up slowly and goes to the sink, starts to run the water.

Carl tries to get comfortable in the padded chair. He reads a chapter about Gandhi, although tonight he feels further removed from the story. He makes a few notes about ideas he wants to insert in his manuscript tomorrow. He says a prayer, struggles to feel him-self in the presence of God, doesn't quite succeed. By the time he gets to bed, she's asleep.

RELATIONSHIPS WITH SPOUSES

People with cancer typically identify their spouses as the most important source of support for dealing with ill-ness.[1] This is especially relevant for men, who are likely to have smaller social networks than women[2] and who are much more likely to say they confide only in their spouses.[3,4] These findings point at the importance of marital relation-ships for men dealing with cancer. When the relationship isn't going well, men are likely to have more adjustment problems.[5] Most of the couples we interviewed in our study were explicit about confronting the challenges of illness together, as a team.[6] Men frequently spoke about how grate-ful they were to their spouses, especially for their reassur-ances about their possible or real impotence. Men who did not receive such reassurances or who had a history of con-flict about sexuality seemed to struggle more. Many men commented that they thought it would be incredibly difficult to go through prostate cancer as a single man.

Cancer often has a huge impact on spouses of patients. Many studies have found that spouses report at least as much distress as do patients.[7,8] It also seems that patients are more likely to receive support from people outside the family than are their spouses.[7] So spouses are clearly key players: their support can be critical to the well-being of their husbands, and they face important personal chal-lenges in dealing with the stresses accompanying a care-giving role.

REFERENCES

1. Neuling, S. J., & Winefield, H. R. (1988). Social support and recovery after surgery: Frequency and correlates of supportive behaviors by family, friends, and surgeon. *Social Science & Medicine, 27*, 385-392.

2. Babchuck, N. (1978). Aging and primary relationships. *International Journal of Aging Human Development, 9*, 186-193.

3. Antonucci, T. C., & Akiyama, H. (1987). An examination of sex differences in social support among older men and women. *Sex Roles, 17*, 737-749.

4. Harrison, J., Maguire, P., & Pitceathly, C. (1995). Confiding in crisis: Gender differences in pattern of confiding among cancer patients. *Social Science & Medicine, 41*, 1255-1260.

5. Rodrigue, J. R., & Park, T. L. (1996). General and illness-specific adjustment to cancer: Relationship to marital status and marital quality. *Journal of Psychosomatic Research, 40*, 29-36.

6. Gray, R. E., Fitch, M., Phillips, C., Labrecque, M., & Fergus, K. (2000). Managing the impact of illness: The experiences of men with prostate cancer and their spouses. *Journal of Health Psychology, 5*, 531-548.

7. Northouse, L. L., Mood, D., Templin, T., Mellon, S., & George, T. (2000). Couples' patterns of adjustment to colon cancer. *Social Science & Medicine, 50*, 271-284.

8. Kornblith, A. B., Herr, J. W., Ofman, U. S., Scher, H. I., & Holland, J. C. (1994). Quality of life of patients with prostate cancer and their spouses. *Cancer, 73*, 2791-2802.

Jed Meets Brad and Steven

Jed is a 55-year-old white gay man, treated one year ago with radiation therapy, currently with no evidence of active disease. He lives alone and is employed as a teacher. Brad is a 58-year-old white gay man, diagnosed five years ago, treated with radiation therapy and now on hormone treatment for metastatic disease. He is unemployed, lives alone, and is a Jehovah's Witness. Steven is a 73-year-old white gay man, on watchful waiting for the past ten years. He lives alone and is a retired accountant.

Jed wonders what in the world he's let himself in for. It seemed like a good idea. You know, a safe place to talk, birds of a feather flocking together, a support group for gay men with prostate cancer. But now there's just him and this plump, fussy old guy in a suit, both watching the door to see if anyone else will show up. Both praying for somebody else to show up. Jed has already tried the chitchat route, but it fizzled out real fast. The guy's name is Steven, he's a retired accountant and, although he didn't say it out loud, he's nervous as hell about being here. Jed complained to him about the two other men who phoned, backing out at the last minute. Steven looked like he wished he'd thought of that.

Jed is surprised at his own nerves. He thought it would be easy. After all the work he's done as an HIV/AIDS support volunteer, he'd have thought that a group like this would be a breeze. But this time it's he that's affected, and his reaction has caught him by surprise. Like he said to that researcher, you don't want to be too open about prostate cancer. Word gets around, and soon everybody might be talking about you. Will they be saying that another person hides behind that hunk of a man with a serious appetite for the good life? Stuff like that.

***

Steven isn't just nervous. He's petrified. He tries to remember what this Jed person said to him on the telephone that convinced him to come and sit in this grungy little cancer society group room. It's not like him to have agreed. He thinks of himself as a loner, someone who mostly keeps to himself. But he was intrigued by the idea of other gay men with prostate cancer. He's never met one before. He knows a couple of straight former co-workers who were diagnosed, but he wonders if there are particular issues for gay men. He can't see why there would be, but he's curious to find out. Or at least he was before he got here. He's not sure he likes the look of Jed. Too flamboyant. Steven spent all those years in the closet, doing everything he could to keep from being fingered as a faggot, including stomping out every effeminate mannerism he could identify. Since he retired, he's more relaxed about it all, but he still finds it disconcerting to run into guys who flaunt their gayness.

***

The door swings open revealing a thin man with bleached blond hair, wearing lots of leather. He's smiling lopsidedly.

"Hi. Sorry I'm late. I sat in the bathtub too long. I'm Brad." He eyeballs the two men, smiling. Inside, he's suspicious, worried. The truth is he got to the building early, before the other two, but then he freaked out and decided he'd better go for a walk and decide if he really wanted to do this. He seems to have decided that he does.

***

"Hi. I'm Jed. We talked on the phone." Brad nods and takes a seat.

"I'm Steven." More nodding.

Silence. Awkwardness. Then Jed takes hold of things.

"So, I had the idea for this meeting after the research interview I had." The other two guys nod. They were also interviewed. "When I found out they were talking to other gay guys, I just thought it might be good to get together and see if we had things in common. I know there's this big prostate support group in the city. I actually called them after I was first diagnosed. And they were very helpful. But I didn't think it would likely work to go to their meetings. At least not if I was going to be truthful about my sexual orientation." He smiles.

Steven smiles back knowingly. That's about the last thing he could imagine himself doing.

Brad leans forward. "I went to the Wellness Center because they started a group for men with prostate cancer. But there were only a couple of meetings, and then it folded. Not enough people."

"How did you like it?" Jed asks.

"To tell you the truth, I was glad it folded. Because there were people there who were a lot worse off than I was. And I felt bad for them. It actually made me feel worse."

"Did they know you were gay?" Steven is curious.

Brad hesitates, but then decides he might as well say it. "No, I didn't think it was important. I actually don't like to think of myself as gay. It's true that my orientation is homosexual, but I've never felt comfortable with it, all my life. I've always fought against it. I was married, I have a daughter, I have two grandchildren."

The other two men nod, pretending to understand. Jed thinking "what a loser." Steven not sure what to think.

Jed steps in again, doing his group facilitator thing. "How about if we each take a few minutes and say a bit about our experiences with prostate cancer?" The other two nod, with some trepidation. Brad clears his throat. He knows from his years in therapy that it's better to get it out than to sit on it.

"When I was diagnosed I thought I'd have surgery. But it was complicated. I'm a Jehovah's Witness, so I wouldn't accept a blood transfusion. The first doctor said he wouldn't operate without blood. I went to another doctor who said he would do it. He was a younger guy, and he said that he did most of his operations without blood. But then he did some other tests, and it was bad news. He said it was too late for surgery, because the cancer had spread outside of the prostate, and that the next best thing would be radiation. So that's what I did."

"What was the radiation like?" Steven asks, knowing that he may yet have to find out for himself.

"It wasn't so bad. But I also went on a clinical trial and was on hormones for three years. And of course you get these hot flashes and they're enough to make you crazy. I got really depressed. I was actually suicidal there for a while." Brad stops suddenly, not sure he wants to go on.

Jed turns to Steven. "Do you want to say what happened to you?"

Steven starts out jittery, words coming out in fits and starts. "I was diagnosed ten years ago, but I decided not to have treatment. I've been watching and waiting for all this time. They said back then that they could do the surgery but it was up to me. I don't like invasive surgery. And from what I understood, it doesn't always work. So I went with the monitoring, and I'm okay with that."

"What does monitoring involve?" Jed has wondered if he should have avoided treatment.

"Mostly it's just having regular PSA tests. But sometimes I have to go for biopsies. I've actually had five of them now. I don't think I'll ever get used to them." He crosses his legs, picks a piece of lint off the cuff of his suit jacket. Unexpectedly, his lips spread into an impish grin.

"Do you want to hear a joke about this?"

Jed groans inside. But Brad smiles. "Go ahead."

"Last time, I said to the doctor who was doing the biopsy that my rectum objects to foreign objects. And he says, 'You don't need to worry about this one, because it's made in Canada."

Polite laughter.

Jed picks up the thread. "I know what you mean about the biopsies being difficult. The first time I had one, the instrument broke, and the procedure ended up taking more than an hour. I was literally in tears on the table."

"Oh, that sounds awful." Steven shakes his head in sympathy. "For me it's never been terribly painful, but it's most certainly been uncomfortable. But as long as the results keep coming back like they have, and I don't have to have treatment, I'll put up with them."

Brad asks, "So you don't really have any problems from the cancer?"

"Well, I didn't get the impotence, which would have been a worry if I'd had the surgery. But I do have a urination problem. It's actually better now, since I started this new medication. I still have to get up very frequently in the night, but at least I don't have to stay up because I can't urinate for an hour or so. That was stressful. And urgency is a problem. It can be extremely awkward. You know, I have to run into places on the street and ask if I can use their washroom."

Brad throws his head back and laughs. "Yeah, tell me about it. I was homebound for a long time. Like I wouldn't even go to a restaurant. Even now I have to be careful. I made sure I went before I came in here, and on my way up the stairs I checked where the washroom was."

Both the others laugh sympathetically. Steven can feel that his breathing is less constricted, more relaxed. Jed thinks, maybe this is going to be all right. But he's aware that it's his turn to speak.

"I had radiation treatment like you did, Brad. I don't like surgery. And they said there was less chance I'd be impotent. I had really wonderful care at the hospital. The doctor made me very comfortable. And she wanted to know my concerns. So I told her about my worries about impotence as a single gay man. I mean, that wasn't unusual for me to talk like that, because I'm very open about being gay. But it was really wonderful to have that taken into consideration and be treated accordingly."

Steven feels his breathing constrict again. He didn't even tell his urologist that he was gay. He's just so used to being private about it that it didn't occur to him. It would frighten him to have the doctor know, to possibly treat him differently, probably worse, maybe use the information against him.

Brad is nodding, but he can't imagine telling his urologist that he's gay. A lot of the people he's really close to don't even know that. Sometimes he gets nervous when he's sitting with someone who knows and then someone who doesn't know comes along. It can be a real juggling act.

Jed is continuing. "The last day of my treatment I walked out of the hospital, and I almost started crying right there in the street, because I was finally taking back control of my life. But what I hadn't realized was that the symptoms would get worse after the treatment ended. About a month later I had bleeding from my rectum. And it's still giving me some problems. I guess what I've realized is that it's not possible to get all the control back. A while back my PSA went up at one of my visits, and I was absolutely stressed out. I had to book off work while I was waiting for the results. It turned out okay, but I couldn't believe how hard that was. The doctor said not to worry so much, but that's easier said than done."

Brad pushes the wave of hair off his forehead. "The funny thing for me is that the diagnosis was almost like a relief. So was the news that the cancer had spread." Both Steven and Jed look at Brad as if he has three heads. "I have this underlying death wish, and it's like having cancer relieves you of the responsibility of doing it."

"Why would you feel that way?" Steven asks. Jed wishes that he hadn't.

"It's because of my religious beliefs. The struggles I've had with being homosexual are way worse than having prostate cancer. Sometimes I just want the struggle to end."

Jed grits his teeth, tries to be patient.

"It's like with my sex life. For years after the cancer diagnosis, I couldn't get an erection. And that was just devastating, because sex has been a big part of my life. But in another way it was kind of a relief not to be able to do it. I have one part that says, oh, sex with men is great and I can really enjoy it. And then I have this other part that says, hey, wait a minute, that's not normal, it's not natural, it's a sin. You know what I mean?"

Steven isn't jittery now, just angry. "I'm very involved with my church, but I'm totally opposed to this Christian-right nonsense. Why would you hold those opinions? You can't win that way."

Brad shrugs his shoulders. "I know. I saw this shrink last year who refused to meet with me after the first time because he said he had no patience with anyone with a fundamentalist Christian belief system who's homosexual. I guess I understand his point. But that's just the way I am."

Jed thinks, "what a loser," but then feels bad about it. It can't be easy to live with such contradictions. He tries another tack.

"Well, it's good you got your erection back eventually. I got mine back, too, but it's still not easy. It's harder to count on it, and that's stressful. I've also been realizing that I'm a lot more careful about sex than I used to be. I'm self-conscious about it." Jed hesitates, unsure how much more he wants to say, but decides that he has a responsibility to be open.

"You know, after the radiation my prostate is about the size of a small pea. So naturally there's very little ejaculation. Now this is something that a straight guy wouldn't understand, but it's different for us. You know how one of the themes from the early HIV education was "on me, not in me." Well, that cultivated a kind of eroticism around ejaculation. So now that it doesn't happen, I worry more about my partner, about whether he's being satisfied. I find that I'm not really looking for a mate any more, as if that's no longer an option."

Steven is interested, never having thought about ejaculation as a problem before. It makes him feel grateful that he's avoided having treatment. He doesn't have worries about sexual performance. Besides, his encounters are formal ones with lovely young guys in massage studios. He isn't looking for long-term relationships.

Jed isn't done yet. "Usually, I prefer to have one lover and then

I'm monogamous. But now I've taken to going to bars and getting physical relief in back rooms. You know, it's more anonymous. And if it's dark they won't see how much you ejaculate. And also in the dark, I'll tend to satisfy the other guy more than myself. So he's happy and I get a bit of play."

Jed is feeling embarrassed and vulnerable to have said so much. Brad can tell Jed is struggling, decides not to say anything about how he thinks that encounters in bars and washrooms are entirely disgusting. Instead he tries to be supportive, shares his own perspective.

"I wouldn't want to get involved with anyone and cause him heartaches or problems. I don't think I'm a very stable person. And eventually my health is going to get worse."

Steven chimes in. "I've lived alone so long that I couldn't stand a relationship and having to adapt. You don't have to feel lonely when you're on your own."

Jed appreciates their efforts, but still feels the sense of loss acutely. He hasn't talked this much about the cancer before. He's beginning to see how much he's been in the closet about it. Which is kind of ironic given that all his friends tease him about having never been in the closet as a gay man. Not many of them know about his struggles with prostate cancer.

"I need to become more positive and accepting." It's Jed trying to summarize his position.

Brad responds. "I think it's hard work to be positive. Like I was saying, I was really depressed for quite a while. Before I was diagnosed, I'd been planning to redo my apartment, like decorate and paint it. But afterwards, I thought, I can't do it. I just don't have the energy. And then I thought, why bother, I'm not going to be around much longer anyway."

He looks at the other guys, decides they really are interested. "When I was depressed someone would ask me how I was, and I'd tell him. And it would sort of bum us both out. So after a while I got to the point where somebody would ask me, and I'd say, 'fine,' no matter how bad things were or what I was going through. I don't even want to talk about it now, because I find it's not a good thing to talk about it. I've found it's better to just do the best you can and push on."

"So do you think it's not good to talk like we've been doing here?" Steven asks.

"No, I think this is okay. Sometimes you have to tell the truth and say what's on your mind. But you can go overboard with it."

Jed reasserts himself. "I don't want to be harping about prostate cancer this and that, forever and ever. That's for sure! But I think it would be good for me to get it more out in the open so that I'm not so paranoid about what other people will think about me."

"Have you told people at work?" Brad asks.

"Some I have. But I've also not told people who care about me. I think I need to change that. What about you, Brad? What have you told the people you work with?

Brad looks down at the carpet, avoiding eye contact. "I haven't been able to work since I was diagnosed. What with fighting the depression and the after-effects of the prostate cancer, I just couldn't cope. They replaced me while I was off on sick leave, and then there was no way to go back. That was the end of my career, so to speak. It's hard sometimes. Because I don't feel like I should have to retire, that my working life should be over. I feel too young to lose all of that."

"I think it's just a matter of getting used to not working," says Steven. "I liked being an accountant, but I'm very happy not to be doing it any more. I think you just get used to a different way of life over time."

Jed smiles, but thinks that it isn't the same for someone like Steven, who must be 70. Then, it might be okay, but not when you're still in your 50s.

The three of them fall into silence. It stretches out. All of them are separately thinking about what's been going on here. All sense that there is something important about what they've been doing. None of them is sorry any more that he made the effort to get here. But each is wondering whether he will do it again.

Later, they talk about what to do next. They all say they might be interested in getting together again, but when they leave, a date has not been set. Will there be another meeting of the gay men's prostate cancer support group?

MEN AND DIVERSITY

Men's experiences with prostate cancer raise different issues for different men, and this variability is related to how men understand masculinity. Too often, research related to prostate cancer, or more broadly to men's health, has focused only on white, middle-class, heterosexual men—largely because these men are easier to recruit into studies. So most of what has been written about men coping with prostate cancer ignores how other men may be affected. Men who are gay, or men who are members of a cultural minority group, experience prostate cancer and masculinity in particular ways that are influenced by their larger life contexts. While some of the experiences of white, middle-class, heterosexual men will be relevant to them, other experiences will not be. In the research used to inform "Jed Meets Brad and Steven," and in Prostate Tales *itself, I've tried to address this issue by including some of the perspectives and experiences of gay and black men.*

I wish to avoid creating the impression that any subgrouping of men has predictable responses to having prostate cancer. It doesn't. For example, while all gay men share certain common issues related to prostate cancer, each individual takes up these issues in very different ways. Similarly, it is a mistake to consider black men as a unified group. And there is also remarkable variability among traditionally masculine white men. The incredible diversity among men must be acknowledged if we are to understand, and help alleviate, the many possible impacts of prostate cancer in men's lives.

Ben Answers the Phone

Ben is a 65-year-old black man diagnosed three months ago and not yet decided about what to do—but leaning towards watchful waiting. He is single and is a manager of a program for homeless people.

The pitcher tugs at his cap, licks the palm of his hand, digs a toe into the mound. He goes into the long wind-up, front leg kicking high, arm flying straight over the top. The camera tracks the ball's path, displaying that it's outside of the strike zone by at least a foot. The Yankee batter flips his bat aside and trots towards first base. Ben groans and digs a meaty hand into the bowl of sour cream and onion chips. He considers shutting the tube off. Having suffered through three blowouts in the last few days, he doesn't know if he can bear to watch the Jays come apart again, especially against these cursed Yankees, so full of themselves and their tradition. He briefly considers his alternatives and decides to leave the TV on and see what happens. Maybe they can get themselves out of this bases-loaded situation. Ha! Until they get some decent pitching, and there's sure no sign of that in sight, it's going to be one groan after another. Not like with those World Series teams. Or even better, when his old buddy George Bell was still in town, smacking the ball out of the park. And taking swipes at the manager and the media and the fans. Now, George knew how to keep things interesting.

The phone rings. Ben scowls at it. Probably another telemarketer. Or, even worse, Joyce calling again to find out why he's been hiding out. But he decides to take the risk and make the effort, thinking it might be Roy wanting to go bowling. He hits the mute button and propels himself off the sagging couch, getting to the phone just before the machine kicks in.

"Yeah."

"This Ben?" He doesn't recognize the voice but figures it must be somebody he knows.

"Yeah, that's me. Who's this?"

"It's Larry Johnson. How are you doing tonight?"

It takes Ben a second to place the name, but then it clicks. It's that know-it-all old geezer always organizing things for the Jamaican community organization. Last time he talked to Larry, he ended up buying a couple of raffle tickets. No way he's going to fall for that again.

"I'm okay, Larry. What can I do for you?"

"I was calling to see if you might want to meet me for a cup of coffee and a piece of cake at Dooney's. It'd be my treat."

Ben doesn't know what to make of this. It's not like he and Larry are old friends. Something's going on, and Ben's pretty sure he's not going to like it.

"Thanks, but I can't get away. I'm expecting company soon...." He produces a deep chuckle. "And she wouldn't want to be stood up."

Larry chuckles back. "No, no. I wouldn't want to get in the way of your action, Ben." His tone turns back to serious. "I was just hoping to have a chat about a topic of mutual interest. Maybe you'd have time later in the week?"

Ben can see that it's not going to be so easy to slip out of this. And, almost against his will, he's starting to get curious.

"Why don't you just say what you have to say?"

There's a pause at the other end. Ben listens to Larry breathing.

"I'd thought it would be better if we could talk in person."

Ben is starting to get riled. And out of the corner of his eye, he watches a Yankee base-runner walk home to score a run.

"I'd rather you spit it out. What's so important that you think you need to butter me up with coffee and cake?"

"Okay. Ben. I can see I'm not doing this very well. Let me get to the point. I'm phoning because somebody told me you have prostate cancer."

Ben feels the bottom fall out of his stomach, is pierced by the now-familiar fear. Then his grip tightens on the phone. He wants nothing more than to reach through the line and strangle this self-important busybody.

"And who told you this?" His tone flat and hard.

"Priscilla. It just came up in conversation. We're on the same union committee at the factory."

Ben exhales loudly.

"What do you mean, it just came up in conversation? Goddamn, I shoulda known better than to tell that sister of mine. She never could keep her mouth shut about anything."

"Listen, Ben, don't be too hard on her. I had prostate cancer myself, and so I was talking about that, and she up and started crying. She said you don't want anyone knowing about your diagnosis, but that she's worried sick about you. So she asked if I'd have a word with you."

Larry's tone is all concerned and reasonable, which only makes Ben madder. He doesn't want this man knowing about his cancer. He has this urge to break things.

"Goddamn women. Always trying to fix everything. I don't really want to talk about this."

"Ben, I thought you might want to hear about my experiences with prostate cancer. I know I found it really helpful to talk with other men who've been through it."

That stops Ben in his tracks. He's been so focused on keeping things hidden, he's never really thought about what other men might know. He decides to go along with it, at least for a minute.

"Okay. So what's it been like?"

"I was lucky. I have a good urologist. He told me to have the surgery and got me in quick for the operation. They took the prostate out, and the cancer's all gone. Just like that."

"Uh, huh." Ben's been to a urologist too. He knows there are other choices besides surgery. And he's pretty much decided on not having any treatment at all. But he doesn't see what business that is of Larry's.

Larry continues. "Surgery's really the only way to cure it. I can't understand why some men choose otherwise. What about you, Ben? What are you going to do?"

Ben's panic starts to rise again. He doesn't want to feel this anymore. And there's something about Larry's tone that makes Ben think that Priscilla has already shared this information. He can see that the only way to deal with this little prick will be to push back.

"The doctor said I could just wait and do nothing if I want. They'll keep checking that the cancer isn't growing. So I don't see why I should volunteer for the knife if doctors don't think it's necessary." Ben figures that should be the end of the conversation, but Larry is right back at him.

"It sounds like you should see another urologist. I can give you the name of mine. You're playing with fire here, Ben. Didn't he explain to you that the cancer can suddenly accelerate and then you only learn about it when it's too late? Cancer kills! God gave us early detection so that we'd have the opportunity to go on living. You can fix this if you do something now. If you don't, there's a good chance you'll end up dead."

Ben doesn't like this talk about dying. Who does this guy think he is to be laying these heavies on him? He strikes back.

"Did I miss something, or did you get a medical degree in your time off from the factory?"

"There's no need to be that way. I'm just trying to help here, Ben. And, yes, I've done a lot of reading about cancer in the last year."

"So if you know so much about prostate cancer, why aren't you saying anything about how it affects sex?" Ben says it aggressively, but part of him is worried about raising the topic, as if maybe it's only he who's making the sex problems into a big thing.

"It doesn't have to be such a problem. I've got my erection back just about as good as it was. They have these new surgical techniques that save the nerves to the penis, and you don't have to end up being impotent."

This is new information for Ben, and it makes him uneasy about his doctor and about his decision. But he doesn't want to trust Larry's information. And he isn't sure that Larry isn't bullshitting him about the impotence piece. He decides to push it further.

"Maybe you're just one of the lucky ones, that is, if you're being straight with me. My doctor said at least two-thirds of men can't get it up after surgery. He said prostate cancer is slow growing and that I'm more likely to die of something else, especially because I have diabetes. So I don't see the point of giving up sex when I don't have to."

Larry loses his concerned and reasonable tone, moves into anger.

"This is just so typical. It's exactly what my doctor said to me. He says he has problems with the black men he sees. White people come to his office, they're diagnosed, they go home and they tell their wives and they come back for surgery. Then they go out and find a drugstore and buy some Viagra and they live happily ever after. But not black people. They come into the office and say, 'Don't tell my wife, please.' They say they want time to think about things, they want to know how long they can possibly wait before treatment. They want to know if there are any herbs that could help them save their erections. And all the time the cancer's growing."

Ben slams his hand on the kitchen counter, can't believe what he's hearing.

"Seems like you're saying that white people are the ones who do things the right way. Well, I think I've heard that before. There's nothing wrong with wanting to have sex. Maybe it doesn't matter to you, but I have a lot of women out there waiting for me." Ben knows he's overstating his case, but it's true he always has had a way with women, and he doesn't want to lose what he has going with Joyce.

Larry is still hot. "Listen, Ben, I've done as much for the Caribbean community as anybody. So don't be saying that I'm against my own people. But I'm just sick of this macho attitude.

Friends of mine have died because they wouldn't face up to the facts. Do you prefer to have an erection or be lying in a coffin? Isn't it better to be alive, even if you pee yourself or you only have five percent of your erection?"

Ben has had just about as much of this as he can take. "You know what, Larry, I'm not sure I want to be wandering around with everybody knowing I'm a eunuch. And maybe I'd rather be dead than lose what's important to me. So why don't you show some respect for other people? And now I am done talking with you about this."

There's a silence that stretches out. Larry breaks it.

"I'm sorry I got you upset, Ben. But I hope you'll change your mind and get an opinion from another doctor. I'd hate to be visiting you next on your deathbed..."

"Larry, I don't want any more of your advice."

"Okay, it's your decision, and I respect your right to do what you think is right. So, all the best, Ben."

"Same to you, Larry."

Ben hangs up. He shakes his head from side to side, fighting off the welling tears. He reaches for the chips with one hand and hits the volume button with the other. He's just in time to catch the score. The Yankees only managed the one run in the eighth. So with the heart of the Jays' lineup coming up in the ninth, maybe there's still a possibility of a comeback....

MAKING TREATMENT DECISIONS

A diagnosis of prostate cancer occurs within a context of medical uncertainty that is unparalleled among other types of cancer. There is no agreement among specialists about the "right" way to treat cancer of the prostate.[1] In the case of localized disease, the relative merits of three primary approaches—(1) the radical prostatectomy; (2) external beam radiation; and (3) watchful waiting—have been vigorously debated.[2] More recently, seed implant radiation (brachytherapy) has also become popular.

Research does not reveal a single approach that would be best for all men. It does suggest that men are more likely to live longer with treatment (than without), but usually with a poorer quality of life. So for men to make decisions, they have to think beyond purely medical issues, to consider their values and preferences. Choices involve trade-offs; the likelihood of more of one thing but less of another. For example, with watchful waiting men have to be able to tolerate knowing that there is cancer in their bodies and that it might suddenly grow and become life-threatening before potentially curative treatment could be introduced. Some men find such inaction intolerable, while others would rather wait than have to deal with the consequences of treatment.

The absence of medical consensus about how to treat prostate cancer means that decision-making becomes an elaborate process for most men. In a study we conducted with men who chose radical prostatectomy as treatment, we found that many were shocked to have so little definitive direction from medical specialists, and they were initially overwhelmed with what was required of them in coming to terms with the information about various options.[3] Although most eventually felt they were in a position to make a good decision, and many found it valuable to have been forced to learn so much about their disease, the process was extremely challenging and time-consuming.

REFERENCES

1. Klotz, L. (2000). *Prostate cancer: A guide for patients.* Toronto: Prospero Books.

2. Warde, P., Catton, C., & Gospodarowicz, M. K. (1998). Prostate cancer: Radiation therapy for localized disease. *Canadian Medical Association Journal, 159,* 1381-1388.

3. Gray, R. E., Fitch, M. I., Phillips, C., Labrecque, M., & Klotz, L. (1999). Presurgery experiences of prostate cancer patients and their spouses. *Cancer Practice, 7,* 130-135.

John Takes a Walk

*John is a 64-year-old white man who had a radical
prostatectomy ten months ago and is currently disease-free. He is married and is a retired union
man.*

"I can't see what the problem is with buying gifts. It's not like
we have a huge family or that there's any of us that can't afford it.
Christmas wouldn't be the same without gifts." Matty stands with
hands on hips, face flushed, glaring at her daughter Ellen. John is sitting at the kitchen table, just out of the line of fire, doing his best to
ignore them. He takes a sip of his coffee, turns the page of his newspaper.

"But, Mom, we're adults now. You'd think there wouldn't be the
same need to do the gift-giving thing." John notices how much
Ellen's voice sounds like his wife's when she's upset. "I think we
should pool our money and send it to Oxfam. That would be more
in the spirit of Christmas."

Matty's right back at her, louder now. "Nobody's stopping you
from giving money to charity. Just don't go imposing your values on
everybody else. Tradition is important, you know, and when you
have kids...." John stops reading, peers over the top of the paper. He
sees Matty's white knuckles clutching the kitchen counter, observes
Ellen's chin jutting forward. He lowers his head.

"Don't start in about my having kids again. Why do you have to
keep bringing that up? I'll have kids when and if it's right for me.
This conversation is about Christmas."

"I'm trying to read here." John knows better, but still the words slip out. He keeps the paper up in front of his face, hoping it will shield him from the predictable consequences.

"Oh, so sorry to interrupt you, Homer Simpson. How thought-less of us to interfere with your leisure by dealing with practical family issues." It's Matty's sarcastic tone, especially dripping for him. Comparing him to a big, dumb, hopeless cartoon character.

He can't leave it alone.

"I don't see why it has to be such a big issue. It wouldn't be a world calamity if we gave gifts or if we didn't give gifts. Why don't you sit down and discuss it like you're members of the same family? Maybe you could compromise; do smaller gifts and also a dona-tion."

Ellen glares at him. "Dad, would you just stay out of it?"

"Yeah." Matty nods vigorously. "All we need is you in your ministerial mode. Why don't you go play golf or something?"

John sighs and returns to reading. He'd like to go play golf, but the guys aren't due to pick him up for another couple of hours. He'll just mind his own business, let them sort it out.

It takes a few minutes, but the women start to make peace. They strike a compromise. It's pretty much the same solution he sug-gested, but he's not about to bring that to their attention.

"So whom should we invite for Christmas dinner this year?" Matty asks Ellen. They have always invited people who don't have other places to go, people who don't fit in. John takes silent pride in this tradition.

"I think Paul will be in town, so let's ask him."

John can't remember which one Paul is. The kids have so many friends. "Is that the homosexual lad that Andrew went to school with?"

"Gay, dad. The term is gay!" They're both staring daggers at him.

"Whatever." He knows he should apologize, but it's not like he means anything bad by it. He's always getting the wrong words. He tries to remember, but, given his years in the navy reserve, and before that growing up in a household of racist rednecks—he thinks it's a miracle he does as well as he does.

Matty turns towards Ellen. "You go ahead and invite Paul. And what about those friends of yours from Pakistan?"

"Omar and Shahina? I'm not sure if they'd want to come, but I'll ask. And what about Sally? Now that she's separated she'll be alone, and I doubt she can afford to go to Vancouver to see her parents."

"Good, I'd love to see her again. That should about do it, don't you think?"

Ellen nods in agreement.

John waits, hoping that they'll think of it on their own. No such luck. He folds his paper and lays it on the table in front of him.

"I think we should invite Uncle Don."

Ellen groans loudly. John feels his face warming.

"I know he's a bit of a bigot, and not all that pleasant to have around all the time, but he is family. And he's just as isolated as the others you want to invite."

Ellen's got her chin out again. "But Dad! He's so offensive. Last time he told those drunken Indian jokes, and poor Nate was sitting next to him. I mean, a member of the anti-racist coalition, and there he was spending Christmas dinner listening to Uncle Don behave like an asshole."

John starts to smile at the memory, ready to concede that it was a slightly unsavory scene. But then Matty takes another cut.

"Don't you think there's enough pomposity in this family without having to add in Don?"

He knows she means him. It's the last straw. His face is hot. He can tell he's seconds away from exploding. He pushes himself out of the chair and strides towards the door.

"I'm going to invite Uncle Don!" It's his old union voice, the one that means there will be no more negotiating on this point. So much for his resolution to stay mellow no matter what. The screen door slams behind him.

He turns left at the foot of the driveway, following the winding road out towards the high school. He knows he'd better walk the long route, give himself plenty of time to cool down. Since he retired he's done this route countless times, mostly when he's been trying to avoid a fight. It's a deliberate decision. He's had too many battles over the years, at home and at work. Fighting with management, with the government, and with the union head office. He wanted to do right by the workers. He believed in what he was doing. Did a good job. Made lots of enemies, lots of friends. But he doesn't want to fight anymore. He's decided it's time to take it easy. Time to enjoy life. Play golf for the fun of it. Cheat like hell because it doesn't matter. He takes his mellowing seriously. He hates it when he gets steamed and loses touch with his intentions.

John's surprised at how he feels so affected by the little spat with Matty and Ellen. Not just the usual pissed off, but also a kind of sad feeling. He's curious about the feeling, doesn't have it very often. Why now?

He hears a car coming up behind him and steps off the road into the grass at the curbside. Stops and looks around. He loves the neighborhood. The old trees, the shaded lawns, the country cottage feel. He's grateful for their good judgement, deciding so many years ago to move out of the city. He steps back onto the road, squints into the rising sun, pulls the brim of his faded red cap further down. Walks on.

He thinks it through. It's part of what he prides himself on, the ability to look at things rationally, in all their complexity. Not at all like Homer Simpson. He decides there are a couple of reasons for the sad feeling. First is that he's out of practice with his role in the family. Everything got disrupted with the prostate cancer diagnosis. Now that things are finally getting back to normal, he's not entirely happy about taking up his old role again.

The second reason seems connected to the interviews he did with that research guy over the past few weeks. It was a bit of a struggle at times. Mostly the interviews were about prostate cancer. He told the guy that it was like a bolt of lightning, right out of nowhere. He had no idea the diagnosis might be coming, didn't even know what a prostate was. After the shock there were intense emotions, unlike anything he could remember. He used a Homer Simpson episode to describe it to the researcher. Homer, whom John admits to adoring, drank some radioactive stuff at work and was supposed to die. First he was in denial, "Ah, you've got the wrong guy!" Then Homer was angry, "I'm madder than hell." Then he broke down and cried for awhile. Finally, there was acceptance, although Homer didn't do so well with that one: "Oh well, we'll get to that someday." He told the researcher guy that he and Homer went through pretty much the same things. They both laughed. The researcher admitted to liking Homer too, which somehow made John feel more at ease.

After the initial roller coaster of emotions, John got serious about finding out what to do. He was shocked that the medical profession seemed to have so little that was definitive to offer. He changed urologists twice, finally found one willing to take the time to answer his questions. He went to the local prostate cancer support group. He surfed the Internet. Got himself on a waiting list for seed implant treatments in Quebec, but there were too many eligibility criteria, and it was taking too long to work out. Finally, after another session with the urologist, he bit the bullet and went for surgery.

Matty was great through that time. So were the kids. They read all the information. Talked pros and cons with him. Made him a priority, curtailed their busy social lives. More than ever before, he talked about what was going on with him to the people around him. He decided he wouldn't be embarrassed about prostate cancer. Sometimes he worried that he talked about it too much.

John arrives at the high school, leans against the wire fence, gazes out over the desolate grounds. Nothing like a schoolyard in summer to give a sense of time passing. It seems like only yesterday that Ellen left the house in her new outfit, ready to brave her first day, and only a few hours ago that he almost choked on the lump in his throat when Andrew gave that speech at his graduation. He's spent a lot of time at this school, volunteering with the athletics program. It all seems hazy now, as if maybe it was some other man who did all that. He backs away from the fence, turns right at the intersection, and starts the loop back towards home, thinking again about prostate cancer.

The surgery went well. No problems, no complications, no infections. All the residents said he was a textbook case. They'd be very surprised if any cancer escaped the prostate gland. But even with that good news, he found the recovery a challenge. He hated being in the hospital. And then he hated being laid up at home. He was so used to being self-reliant, and there he was, incontinent and not even able to tell when he was whizzing. Dealing with the god-damn catheter and then having to restrict himself to no more than one beer at a time. Things gradually improved. Now he's pretty much okay except he can't drink beer and play golf at the same time. He's made that into a running gag with his golfing buddies. Impotence is another story. He keeps that pretty quiet. But it's not a new thing for him, been that way for more than ten years, from way before the prostate cancer. That's another thing that was embarrassing to admit in the interview with the researcher, trying to explain why he didn't do anything about the impotence for all those years. It's not like he didn't want sex. It was embarrassing to admit he was just too embarrassed to try to figure it out. Somehow it's easier now that he has a legitimate reason for the impotence.

The really hard part about the recovery period after the surgery was depending on other people. It was quite a shock for him. He tried to be patient, tried to be gracious. Succeeded sometimes; other times, forget it. Matty was in her element out buying him new underwear and pants. And for the first time they actually talked about what they might do about the impotence. He surprised himself further, said yes to the urologist when he asked John to talk with a couple of men to help them prepare for the prostatectomy.

He feels pretty good about how he's handled the prostate cancer and about how he's communicated about it. But still, he knows it hasn't been enough for Matty, that she hoped for more openness from him, more emotional display. He knows he can't give her what she wants. Part of him is sorry about that, and part of him wishes she would just let him be the way he is.

It's not that he wanted the recovery period to go on and on. It was damned difficult, and he's so relieved to be mobile again. But still, there was something good about having a different routine and having his attention occupied in new ways. And somehow it seemed to improve things in the family. Tensions eased for a while. He stopped his Homer imitation. People stopped expecting it of him. No wonder it's seemed like a mixed blessing that they're all slipping back into familiar ways.

The last time they met, the researcher guy asked him what it felt like to be interviewed. John said that it had been hard at times. He admitted that he hadn't really wanted to do it in the beginning and only agreed for the good of the cause. But then he said that it had turned out to be kind of a revelation for him. He thought that everyone with prostate cancer could probably benefit from this kind of discussion.

He rounds the last bend in the road and sees the blue Olds in the drive. He picks up his pace, checks his watch. Fred is early to pick him up. That's all right with John, because he's goddamn well ready for a good game of golf. He breaks into a grin. He plans to enjoy himself and cheat like hell.

RECOVERING FROM TREATMENT

The first few months following treatment for prostate cancer can be a challenging time. Very often, men are unprepared for what they will face.[1,2] Sometimes this is because they don't get enough information from health professionals; sometimes it's because they have trouble taking in the information that is offered to them. After surgery, men (and their spouses) often have difficulties dealing with catheter care, post-operative pain, fatigue, and incontinence.[1] After a course of radiation treatment, patients usually experience fatigue, rectal discomfort, diarrhea, and an urge to urinate frequently.

We found in our study that men were keen to get active as soon as they could after treatment. They equated recovering their physical capacity with taking charge of themselves and their lives again. Sometimes they overexerted themselves. Often tensions arose between husbands and wives about whether the man might be overdoing. Men were often irritable when their typically unrealistic expectations for speedy recovery were not met.[1]

In general, the post-treatment period creates numerous stresses for husbands and wives, requiring considerable patience and negotiation. Sometimes there is also a new kind of intimacy that emerges. But for most couples these changes are temporary disruptions. As the men regain their mobility, they (and their wives) resume their lives and put illness and treatment behind them as much as they can. While this can never be perfectly accomplished, most couples dedicate themselves to minimizing the impact of the disease and getting on with life.[3]

REFERENCES

1. Phillips, C., Gray, R. E., Fitch, M., Labrecque, M., Fergus, K., & Klotz, L. (2000). The early post-surgery experiences of prostate cancer patients and their spouses. *Cancer Practice, 8,* 165-171.

2. Moore, K. N., & Estey, A. (1999). The early post-operative concerns of men after radical prostatectomy. *Journal of Advanced Nursing, 29,* 1121-1129.

3. Gray, R. E., Fitch, M., Phillips, C., Labrecque, M., & Fergus, K. (2000). Managing the impact of illness: The experiences of men with prostate cancer and their spouses. *Journal of Health Psychology, 5,* 531-548.

Frederick Tries for a Job

*Frederick is a 62-year-old white gay man who had
a radical prostatectomy four years ago and is currently disease-free. He lives alone, is unemployed,
and has severe urinary incontinence.*

Frederick wakes in a panic. In the dream he'd been back in
Warsaw, a young man again. He was in one of the grand old theatres,
and the play was *Henry IV*, or at least it started out that way. In the
way of dreams, it unexpectedly shifted to a French farce and then
back to *Henry IV*. Karl was there, beautiful Karl, whom he hadn't
thought about in years. Of course they were arguing. About the
sleeves being too billowy, or maybe not billowy enough. And then
about the stockings and whether he'd chosen the "just right" shade
of blue. The actor, a reluctant model, was turned away, looking
backstage, trying his best to ignore them. But then—and this is when
the panic started—the actor turned upstage towards Frederick, face
flushed red under the bright lights.

"What have you done?!" he bellowed, pointing down at the dark
circle spreading outwards from the crotch of his silken ivory pants.
And then Karl was yelling too.

"You forgot the diapers, you idiot. What kind of costume
designer would forget the diapers?!"

Frederick lies quietly in his bed, letting his heartbeat slow,
relaxing his clenched hands. It was such a long time ago, that life in
Warsaw. Karl and Alex and Darroch and all of the others. The mam-
moth productions and being well paid. And before that the student

days at the Academy of Fine Arts. And before that being with his mother in the theatre, absorbing her love of it all. Such a long time ago. But he shouldn't think about it. The move to Canada had been for the best. It's stupid to romanticize the past. And, besides, he has to get up. It's an important day.

He slides his hand along the bed sheet, checking. Dry! He feels his lips move into a tiny smile. It's now more than six months since a wet morning. Thank God for small mercies! If He would just extend His mercy beyond the horizontal, include the vertical. Another smile, this time at his own irreverence, his endless attempts to manipulate God into behaving properly.

He walks briskly to the toilet. Sits, waits, and is quickly rewarded. He showers and shaves. Then he goes to the closet, opens a new package of diapers. He puts one pair on and stuffs three more into his ancient leather briefcase.

All three pairs of pants, black in case of leaks, are pulled out for inspection. Frederick frowns at them, noting the fraying, the places where his mending is visible. He finally chooses and then turns to shirts. The navy one is newer and more business-like than the pale yellow, so it's no contest. He definitely wants to be conservative and respectable today, the kind of man you'd want to hire to be part of your department store team. He checks that there are no wrinkles. The tie is silver and gray, ten years old now, a remnant from when he had a job he loved. Before downsizing. Before prostate cancer.

He won't be able to go through his whole routine this morning. But coffee is a must. As always, he proceeds with brewing himself a pot while simultaneously admonishing himself for drinking the stuff. Coffee only makes things worse, and it takes up too much of his meager welfare money. His compromise has been to buy the cheaper brands, save the Starbucks blends for special occasions. He will allow himself only one cup this morning, not wanting to fill his bladder.

He sips the barely adequate brew while re-reading Saturday's want ads. The most promising ones have already been marked with his fine-point pen, but he checks that none were missed. He hasn't sent out all the resumes yet, needing first to make sure there will be enough for food and a new supply of diapers before buying more paper. He definitely doesn't want to make that mistake again.

Frederick has already decided to walk, having plotted his route last night. Public transportation is no longer an option except in an emergency. Too many people, too much money, and too many opportunities for embarrassment. He peers out of the single window, notes the fresh snow, the way that the cars spray slush as they pass by in front of the rooming house. He tucks his pants firmly into galoshes, sighs deeply before donning the heavy old brown overcoat, trying not to think how it will look to a prospective employer.

Out on the sidewalk, he's pleased to find it's not as cold as he expected. When the sun gets higher, there could even be some serious melting. Maybe it's a harbinger of spring. The smile springs again to his lips, an acknowledgement of self-deceit, the ridiculousness of hope for Canadians in the first week of February.

"Hi, Frederick." The greeting startles him.

"Oh, hi, Peter. A lovely day, don't you think?"

"Yeah, it's good to see the sun again. I haven't seen you around much lately."

"I've been busy looking for work. I'm on my way right now to an interview." He wonders if it's his imagination, or if Peter looks skeptical.

"Well, good luck with that. Let's get together for coffee some time."

Frederick nods, smiles, and makes to move on.

"Sure. See you."

He turns the corner at the lights and heads towards downtown, thinking about Peter. Coffee might be nice some time, but not for at least a couple of weeks. Nothing against Peter, but he hasn't felt much like company lately. To be truthful, he hasn't felt like company for quite a long while. Pavel, his only real friend, has been after him to be more social. But Frederick tells him he doesn't mind the isolation. That he's always been a bit of a loner. And now, well, there doesn't seem to be as much to say to other people. And when he does talk, the words spill out too fast. Sometimes it seems like he won't be able to stop them.

As the blocks pass, he is getting warm and wishes he had a lighter coat. Then he feels it, the wetness in his groin. It was expected. He always pees more when he's nervous. Still, there's always, like today, that moment of anger, the brief rebellion against the way things are. But thinking that way is a dead-end street for sure, not to be pursued. He deliberately turns his mind away from his skin.

Where was he? Oh, yes, thinking about relationships. It's not as if he's a hermit. He does go and have dinner with Pavel and his wife every few months. And there are a couple of other friends who invite him to their homes, and once in a while he goes. And as for sexual relationships, he had mostly given up on them before the surgery anyway. It's ironic, he thinks, that he can still get an erection. Mind you, it's not as good as it used to be. He smiles. It used to be excellent. But how many men treated for prostate cancer would re-mortgage their houses to have what he has? Lots, he would bet. It almost seems shameful for him to let it go to waste. But, then, other men don't have to deal with his incontinence.

He tries not to let his mind go where it wants to go, back along the well-worn grooves of what-ifs and if-onlys. If he had gone to the big teaching hospital instead of the local community hospital. If he had chosen a different surgeon, one who wasn't so old, who didn't wear glasses, who hadn't already done two other surgeries that day. Maybe he should have gone for radiation treatment or done nothing at all and just waited to see if the miniscule tumor would grow. But everyone agreed that surgery would be best, and it made sense to him at the time, and it doesn't do any good to second-guess himself now. That was four years ago.

He knows that he was as prepared as he could have been for the surgery. He'd gotten himself in top shape, worked hard on strengthening those muscles. And he was up walking the day after surgery, eager to recuperate. They told him the flooding was only temporary, would correct itself over time. They were wrong. He saw specialists, did other exercises, made small improvements. By the end of the first year, he had stopped peeing the bed every night and had gotten some of the control back over releasing gas. He tried to stay positive. At least he was free of cancer.

When he talked to that researcher a few weeks back, he said that he didn't blame anyone for what happened, that he respected doctors, but that he just wondered if things could have been different. But later he was suddenly angry, very angry. A whole day of ranting and raving inside his head. He doesn't want to feel that way. What good does it do? He wonders now about whether he should cancel the next meeting with the researcher.

Maybe he should go for more surgery for the incontinence, like the most recent specialist suggests. But he's afraid. Things might get worse instead of better. He knows there are no guarantees with any of this. And, besides, going for surgery would interfere with his finding work, or, if all goes well, with his job.

He's been walking 40 minutes and has come to the shopping mall where he will change. He finds the washroom, cleans himself up, puts on the new diaper. Luckily, none of it leaked through, and his pants are fine. Thank God for small mercies.

It's a five-minute walk from here to the department store, but he has 15 minutes yet before his appointment. He can take his time and reflect on the upcoming interview. He knows he's qualified, having done the same type of work for a dozen years at another store. But now, and here his thoughts take a nasty turn, he's 62 and hasn't worked since before his prostate cancer, hasn't even had an interview in over a year. That despite the hundreds of applications he sent out, the countless cold calls.

There was actually that one job since his illness, but he doesn't want to think about it, especially now. He tries to distract himself. Thinks about going out for coffee after the interview. Starts to go over his mental list of food to buy on the way home. But the memory insists, forces itself to center stage.

It was a garment shop on Spadina, and he was hired as a cutter, about a year after his surgery. Of course he was good at it. The embarrassed owner admitted as much several days after he started. But it was all the trips to the washroom. And, frankly, the smell. Co-workers had complained. Maybe if he had his own room to work in, it would have been okay. But that was not possible here. Frederick didn't argue. He was aware of the looks, of the way people were avoiding him. And back then he hadn't been able to control his gas. He understood. But he was still upset, still went out and got terribly drunk.

Frederick notices that his pace has slowed, that he has almost come to a stop. He is having trouble getting his breath. And he is no longer warm but unbearably hot. He looks at his watch, is alarmed to see he has only a few minutes left before the appointment. He wills his reluctant legs to move more quickly, is grateful when they respond.

He passes through the revolving front door at one minute to the hour, sees the sign at the foot of the escalator and starts in that direction, seeking the personnel department. Then he feels it. The warm wet. Not just in the groin but down his left leg. And then his right leg. He lowers his head and looks. Even the black can't hide the stain.

For a few moments he stands quietly in the foyer, looking around him at the displays in the windows. A couple of them strike his fancy, very much like the kind of work he would do. Then he steps back through the revolving door, out onto the snowy street.

URINARY INCONTINENCE

The vast majority of prostate cancer patients choosing radical prostatectomy experience urinary incontinence, to greater or lesser degrees. In our interviews with men, we found that most were getting their incontinence under control a couple of months post-surgery. But they recalled the earlier indignity and embarrassment of having to wear thick pads, and concerns about dribbling. And we heard numerous stories of inappropriately shaped diapers and unfortunate messes. The men would have appreciated more information from health professionals about what to expect and how to deal with incontinence.[1]

Incontinence in the long term is a more serious matter, one that frankly scares most men. We interviewed men waiting for prostate cancer surgery and found that they were considerably more worried about the possibility of incontinence than they were about the possibility of impotence.[2] And the men were greatly relieved when they were finally able to regain control in the months following surgery. But not everyone regained such control. Some continued to have ongoing dribbling problems, especially if they had a sudden physical stress. A few others had virtually no control at all. Recent studies have reported that most men (70% or more) return to being fully continent by a year post-treatment.[3] Of those with ongoing incontinence problems, a lower proportion (less than 10%) of men retained no control compared to those who experienced intermittent "stress incontinence."[4,5] A variety of interventions are used to treat incontinence, including drug treatments, pelvic floor rehabilitation through behavior therapy, manipulation of the gracilis muscle, and surgical implanting of an artificial urinary sphincter.[3]

REFERENCES

1. Phillips, C., Gray, R. E., Fitch, M., Labrecque, M., Fergus, K., & Klotz, L. (2000). The early post-surgery experiences of prostate cancer patients and their spouses. *Cancer Practice, 8,* 165-171.

2. Gray, R. E., Fitch, M., Phillips, C., Labrecque, M., Klotz, L. (1999). Presurgery experiences of prostate cancer patients and their spouses. *Cancer Practice, 7,* 130-135.

3. Hassouna, M. M., & Heaton, J. P. W. (1999). Prostate cancer: Urinary incontinence and erectile dysfunction. *Canadian Medical Association Journal, 160*, 78-86.

4. Goldenberg, S. L, Ramsey, E. W., & Jewett, M. A. S. (1999). Prostate cancer: Surgical treatment of localized disease. *Canadian Medical Association Journal, 159*, 1265-1271.

5. Stanford, J. L., Feng, Z., Hamilton, A. S., Gilliland, F. D., Stephenson, R. A., Eley, J. W., Altbertsen, P. C., Harlan, L. C., & Potosky, A. L. (2000). Urinary and sexual function after radical prostatectomy for clinically localized prostate cancer: The prostate cancer outcomes study. *Journal of the American Medical Association, 283*, 354-360.

Norm Downs a Few Drinks

Norm is a 63-year-old white man treated six years ago with a radical prostatectomy, now receiving radiation therapy because of evidence of disease recurrence. He is an independent businessman on the brink of a divorce.

Frank picks up the rag and runs it along the length of the bar counter. Then he runs it back the other direction. It's not that there's anything that needs wiping up, more that he's gotten restless. There's only so much TV rugby that he can take at one time, and he's long past that threshold. He'd considered changing the station, but a couple of regulars have their eyes glued to the set. And on a slow day like this, he can't afford to lose any from his handful of patrons. He thinks about reading some of the Dave Robicheaux mystery but doesn't want to devour the whole novel in one gulp, wants to draw the pleasure out over time. He thinks about having another cigarette, but he's already had more than his daily allotment.

The door opens and Norm steps inside, looking pale and haggard. Not the usual Norm, although he's dressed in the usual way, expensive businessman duds. Norm drapes his trench coat over a barstool, places his briefcase on top.

"Hey, Frank, how're you doing?" It's Norm's usual friendly, sincere tone.

"Not bad. How about you, Norm?"

"I'm okay." But the tone slips, and Frank doesn't believe him. "You'd better set me up with a double." Now Frank knows something is wrong. Norm heads towards the washroom at the back of the bar.

Frank can't remember Norm ordering a double before. Usually it's one or at most two Scotches, sipped slowly. But then he remembers the incident, must be ten years ago. He'd forgotten about it because it was so out of character for Norm, getting that plastered, picking fights with two of the other regulars. Later Norm had been effusive in his apologies, paid for all the damage and then some. But it had been quite an evening, one of the rare times he'd had to call the cops. God, Frank hoped he wasn't in for another night like that.

He tries to remember what set Norm off that time. He knows that he was going on and on about it, but a bartender doesn't always listen that closely. It was something about a fight with his teenage son. Maybe the kid took a poke at the old man and then lit out on his own. Something like that.

Then it occurs to Frank that if Norm's upset it probably has to do with the cancer. He doesn't know why he didn't think of it right away. A couple of weeks back Norm was in early, and Frank asked, in his usual interested barkeep style, what he had on for the day. And Norm told him he was on his way to get a radiation treatment for prostate cancer. Frank was shocked, said he had no idea that Norm had been diagnosed. And then he was even more shocked, because Norm told him that he was actually diagnosed five or six years ago and had surgery then, and that he was only having the radiation now because the cancer had spread. Frank felt like shit for asking. And he was amazed yet again about how these guys he thinks he knows go for years talking his ear off but saying dick all about what's really going on in their lives.

Frank had said he was real sorry to hear the news about the cancer.

Norm had leaned over the bar with a glint in his eye and said, "You know what the worst of it is?" Frank said he didn't know, thinking that he wasn't sure he wanted to know. "Well, every damn suit I've got has holes in it from that radiation."

Frank had stared at him for a minute, only slowly realizing he was being had. Then he said the first thing that came into his head. "You haven't got anything a fire extinguisher wouldn't cure. You let me know if you need any help with that." And then they'd had a bit of a laugh and Norm had left and neither of them had mentioned the cancer since.

Now, Norm is back from the washroom, not looking like he's in a joking mood today. Frank decides to wipe the bar at the other end. But it doesn't take long before Norm is asking for another double.

"Today's a special day for me." Norm says it with bravado.

"Oh, yeah, how's that Norm?"

"I just got served with divorce papers."

"No kidding. You've been married a long time, haven't you?"

"Forty-two years. It's a bit of a shocker. If she was going to leave me, I thought she would've done it long ago. The timing isn't so great, what with my having to deal with the cancer right now."

"Yeah, really. That's tough."

"Oh, I don't blame her. She should have kicked me out long ago."

"Uh huh." Frank is noticing that one of the rugby fans is looking at him like he's thirsty. "I've got to take an order. Back in a minute."

"Before you go, set me up another, would you?"

"You should think about going a bit slow with the Scotch." Frank gives the warning but sets up the drink anyway. From the look Norm is giving him, he can tell he's not in the mood to be taking advice.

Frank takes a bottle of beer over to the rugby fan's table, thinking as he goes about what Norm has said so far. He doesn't know the wife, and Norm has never said anything about her that Frank can remember. But he does know that some of the other regulars don't much like Norm. And that there were ripples a couple of times about Norm maybe banging other men's wives. Once a guy had come into the bar looking for Norm when he wasn't there, a guy with a head of steam going. So maybe Norm had this coming.

Once Frank's back behind the bar, Norm waves him over.

"You know, I've had a thing for women since I was a kid. Never could stay away from them. I got started when I was 13. Learned about the birds and the bees from the street and from actual practical use."

"So you had some fun, did you?" Teenage sex is a bit of a sore point for Frank. Having grown up in a conservative religious family, he's sure he didn't get his fair share.

"Yeah, when I was 15 my buddy and I worked one summer on an army base. Come the weekend we'd go and find the M.O. and we'd sit down in front of his desk and say we needed condoms. He'd want to know how many, and we'd say about six each. And we'd go to the little village nearby and use them all up. We would have maybe three different girls each on the weekend, but sometimes we'd have the same girl, the two of us."

Frank doesn't entirely believe the story, knowing that men are such bullshitters when it comes to sex. But he suspects it might be at least partly true. He decides to find out more.

"So what do you attribute your success with women to?" It comes out sounding slightly sarcastic, but Norm doesn't notice. Too far into the booze for fine discriminations.

"Oh, I learned early on that if you have a decent kind of patter and put it forward in an adventurous way, or express some interest or fondness for women, then they usually reciprocate." Norm struggles to get the last word out. Points at his glass. Frank sighs and pours the drink.

"It's all about saying the right thing at the right time. And being courteous. And most of all...." He stops and looks at Frank, big goofy grin spread on his face.

"What?"

"You have to know how to dance. I never met a girl who didn't like to dance."

"Right." Frank is irritated. He never learned to dance until he went to college. Was always awkward about it.

"So what does this have to do with your divorce?" Frank thinks that his question should sober Mr. Cassanova up a bit. And he's right. The grin disappears.

"You know, when you've had a lot of partners before you get married, you tend to want to carry on that kind of lifestyle after you're married. So that's what I did. And I'm not proud of it at all." He actually hangs his head, drifts into silence.

Frank is just about to wander off when Norm's head jerks upright again. "The thing is that about 48 percent of women are unorgasmic." Frank is pretty sure Norm has made up the number, but he's learned better than to ask a serious drinker for corroboration. And, besides, Norm has more to say.

"When you're in the position where you're married to somebody who's unorgasmic and you've had lots of fellatio and cunnilingus...." Norm stops, takes a deep breath after the effort of getting those words out, "...it's hard not to go looking for more. Maybe if you didn't have that experience, maybe you wouldn't worry about it." Norm's slurring now, and Frank resents the possible implication that he could be one of the guys who wouldn't know that he was missing anything.

"So you think you were just a victim of your past experience, is that it?" Frank knows he's living dangerously. Norm gives him a bleary stare, teetering on the edge of belligerence. He pulls himself back from the brink.

"No, there's more to it than that. Men need adventure in their lives. And when you're in business, a lot of the work is mundane and repetitive, so extramarital interests keep you going. There's excitement in the chase. And excitement in getting away with something. And when the woman's younger, there's a big rush in being able to sweep her off her feet. You know, it makes you feel really alive."

Frank nods sulkily. Things haven't been all that great between him and Margie lately. He's thought about having an affair but knows it's not what he really wants. And he doesn't want to start going to hookers again. Mostly, he just wishes things were better with Margie.

"So what you're saying is that it's perfectly natural for men to have affairs, especially if their wives aren't adventurous enough?" Now Frank sounds outright hostile.

Norm looks Frank straight in the eye, suddenly not bleary at all. "Up yours."

Their eyes stay locked. Finally, Norm looks down. His tone softens.

"I never said I wasn't to blame. It's just that now I was finally ready to settle down with her. It's not like I don't love her, you know. And with this cancer treatment, my addiction to sex is finally over."

"Oh." Frank suddenly remembers reading something about prostate cancer, about how it can ruin your sex life. What a drag for Norm. He's surprised to feel some sympathy.

Norm smiles wearily. "Actually her timing is perfect. She waited until I really needed her before taking her revenge. It's what I deserve."

He gets off his stool unsteadily. Goes to grab his briefcase.

"Can I call you a cab, Norm? You shouldn't drive."

Norm breaks into a smile. "Thanks, but a walk will do me good."

"Listen, I'm sorry I got a bit provocative back there."

"Hey, not to worry. What's a few words between old friends like us?" Frank's glad to hear the old cheerful tone back in Norm's voice. Even if he doesn't believe it. Even if he never believes it again.

"Goodnight, Norm."

"Goodnight, Frank."

The door bangs shut.

ERECTILE DYSFUNCTION (IMPOTENCE)

The loss or compromising of penile erections is a common consequence of prostate cancer treatment. Prostatectomy, and to a lesser degree radiation treatment, damages the complex of nerves and/or blood vessels responsible for erections.[1,2] Hormonal therapy typically results in drastically reduced sexual desire, making matters worse.[3]

Impotence appears to be more likely to occur with sur-

gery than with external beam radiation therapy, and least likely to occur with brachytherapy (seed implant radiation).[4] But the dysfunction men face has been difficult to pin down. In a recent U.S.-population-based study, 60% of men treated with radical prostatectomy were impotent 18 months after surgery.[5] Other studies have shown similar or higher rates.[2,6,7] Attempts have been made in recent years to minimize damage during surgery through "nerve-sparing" techniques.[8] While this clearly can offer benefits, discrepancies exist in the literature regarding the degree of improvement for sexual functioning with this approach relative to the standard procedure.[9] For external beam radiation therapy, the authors of one recent review paper estimated that at least half of men become impotent following treatment,[10] while early results from studies of brachytherapy are suggestive of substantively lower rates.[11]

What is also important to acknowledge is that many research reports about erectile dysfunction following prostate cancer treatment focus only on the total incapacity to produce erections. While this gives one perspective on the seriousness of the topic, it obscures the experiences of men who retain some limited capacity. Findings from our study of couples showed that most of these men also had major challenges to face in dealing with their reduced and uncertain capacity.[12] Treatment for prostate cancer rarely allows a return to normal pre-illness sexual functioning.

There are various pharmacological and technological treatments for erectile dysfunction, including injections of medications into the penis, transurethral suppositories, oral agents (including Viagra), vacuum pumps, and penile prostheses. All of these treatments have some proven degree of effectiveness, but their usefulness to individual men is very unpredictable. In our study with couples, we heard more stories of failure than of success, and we discovered that men had not anticipated how difficult the technologies would be to use, nor how often they would turn out to be unsuccessful.[12]

It is critical to make the distinction between impotence and libido. Impotence refers to the inability to get or maintain erections. Libido refers to the desire to have sex. While some men suffer from both impotence and lack of libido, it is common to have one and not the other. Following surgery or radiation, many men have difficulties getting erections but have every bit as much desire as in the past. But men on hormone treatments usually lose their desire, although some may still be able to get erections (either naturally or with the assistance of aids).

How bothered are men by the sexual problems that often follow prostate cancer treatment? Evidence from our own and other studies suggests that this varies enormously, partly due to differences in age and in the previous importance given to sex in men's lives. In one large study of men treated with prostatectomy, 42% reported sexuality to be a "moderate" to "severe" problem.[5] In our work, we found that most men downplayed the possible impact of sexual changes in the periods leading up to and immediately following initial treatment. But a year later, many were feeling that impact much more acutely, with some men struggling a lot.[12]

REFERENCES

1. Hassouna, M. M., & Heaton, J. P. W. (1999). Urinary incontinence and erectile dysfunction. *Canadian Medical Association Journal, 160,* 78-86.

2. Robinson, J. W., Dufour, M. S., & Fung, T. S. (1997). Erectile functioning of men treated for prostate cancer. *Cancer, 79,* 538-544.

3. Schover, L. R. (1993). Sexual rehabilitation after treatment for prostate cancer. *Cancer (Suppl.), 71,* 1024-1030.

4. Shrader-Bogen, C. I., Kjelberg, J. L., McPherson, C. P., & Murray, C. L. (1997). Quality of life and treatment outcomes: Prostate carcinoma patients' perspectives after prostatectomy or radiation therapy. *Cancer, 79*, 1977-1986.

5. Stanford, J. L., Feng, Z., Hamilton, A. S., Gilliland, F. D., Stephenson, R. A., Eley, J. W., Altbertsen, P. C., Harlan, L. C., & Potosky, A. L. (2000). Urinary and sexual function after radical prostatectomy for clinically localized prostate cancer: The prostate cancer outcomes study. *Journal of the American Medical Association, 283*, 354-360.

6. Heathcote, P. S., Mactaggart, P. N., Boston, R. J., Carl, A. N., Thompson, L. C., & Nicol, D. L. (1998). Health-related quality of life in Australian men remaining disease-free after radical prostatectomy. *Medical Journal of Australia, 168*, 78-86.

7. Talcott, J. A., Rieker, P., Clark, J. A., Propert, K. J., Weeks, J. C., Beard, C. J., Wishnow, K. I., Kaplan, I., Loughlin, K. R., Richie, J. P., & Kantoff, P. W. (1998). Patient-reported symptoms after primary therapy for early prostate cancer: Results of a prospective cohort study. *Journal of Clinical Oncology, 16*, 275-283.

8. Klotz, L. (2000). *Prostate cancer: A guide for patients.* Toronto: Prospero Books.

9. Fergus, K., Gray, R. E., & Fitch, M. (2002). Sexual dysfunction and the preservation of manhood: Experiences of men with prostate cancer. *Journal of Health Psychology, 7*, 303-316.

10. Warde, P., Catton, C., & Gospodarowicz, M. K. (1998). Radiation therapy for localized disease. *Canadian Medical Association Journal, 159*, 1381-1388.

11. Davis, W., Kuban, D. A., Lynch, D. F., et al. (2000). Quality of life after radical prostatectomy vs. brachytherapy for localized prostate cancer. *Journal of Urology, 163*, 286-292.

12. Gray, R. E., Fitch, M. I., Phillips, C., Labrecque, M., & Fergus, K. (2002). Prostate cancer and erectile dysfunction: Men's experiences. *International Journal of Men's Health, 1*, 5-20.

Doug Goes Fishing

Doug is a 66-year-old white man who had a radical prostatectomy 14 months ago and is currently disease-free. He is semi-retired, married, and has a history of depression.

"I think I'll have one more of those sandwiches, dear. What have you got left?" Doug winks at Lucille. She smiles in return, sweeping back the gray strand that keeps blowing across her face. She reaches for the picnic basket, peers in.

"Well, let's see. Looks like there's a tuna and mayonnaise and a peanut butter and banana."

Tommy is ignoring them, eyes fixed on the end of his rod, as if by staring hard enough he can will it to bend, can make a trout leap for a lure somewhere back behind the boat.

"Maybe I'll try the peanut butter and banana. It can't be as bad as it sounds." Doug keeps his tone matter-of-fact, testing the waters.

"Grandpa!" Tommy takes the bait. He twists his small frame towards Doug, brown eyes flashing. "You don't even like peanut butter. You're just trying to make trouble. Isn't he, Grandma?"

Lucille chuckles.

"You're right about that, Tommy. Your grandpa is a troublemaker from way back."

Tommy giggles.

"Yeah, he should watch me so he can learn how to behave." He giggles again, clearly delighted by the idea of being a model for good behavior.

"I'm not so sure about that." Lucille shakes her head from side to side, posing as contemplative. "It strikes me that you and your grandfather are a lot alike on that score. Both born troublemakers."

The boys look at each other. Doug rolls his eyes. They laugh in unison. There's nothing boys like better than making trouble and being loved for it.

Lucille hands the peanut butter sandwich to Tommy, the tuna to Doug. There was never really any doubt about who would get which one, or for that matter who would go without. She's thinking how she needs to lose weight anyway. And how it's so good to see Doug happy again. She can't believe how well he's doing. She's still recovering from having her world destroyed when Doug got depressed, long before the prostate cancer diagnosis. She's not sure if she could manage another bout of that terrible darkness.

Doug steers the skiff into a bay, peering intensely for any partially submerged logs. Satisfied that it's safe, he lets his gaze rise to the rocky shoreline. The forest is thick right down to the water. Several of the birches are stripped of bark at the bottom. He points and Tommy's eyes follow his finger eagerly.

"Beavers."

Tommy nods his agreement and then scans the bay, hoping to spot one.

Doug watches the boy's curly head turn, struck again by how much he looks like Doug's son, Tommy's father, at the same age. It's not an entirely happy association, stirring tentacles of worry in his chest. What will happen if his son and daughter-in-law go ahead with the divorce? Will Tommy be even more neglected by his father? Would it help to talk with his son? Or would he just erupt in anger again, shouting that Doug was a fine one to talk. Doug could only agree with him, say he's sorry, say he wishes he had been a different kind of father.

Doug doesn't want to think about this any more. He looks up.

"Why don't you read some more, Lucille?"

She's brought the Rudyard Kipling compilation, not wanting to fish herself and knowing Tommy will need extra stimulation to make the waiting easier.

"Okay, but not until I finish my tea. Would you like me to read again, Tommy?"

"Sure, Grandma."

Doug eases up on the throttle as they leave the bay. It's choppier now, so he's keeping them close to shore.

Tommy is sprawled across the wooden seat, head resting on the oarlock, waiting for the fish to come. Grandpa had a bite about an hour back. And they've been jumping around the boat. So he knows they're out there, assumes with a boy's confidence that it's just a matter of time. He wants to catch the first one, before Grandpa does.

Tommy feels good. The stampede at Williams Lake yesterday was awesome. Ditto with the mountain sheep down by the highway. And best of all so far was sitting with Grandpa in the car in the dark, waiting for the black bears to visit the dump. He didn't really believe they would come, but come they did. And while they were waiting, Grandpa told him hunting stories from when he was young, a hundred years ago. He wanted to stay there all night watching the bears and listening to Grandpa, but then he went and fell asleep and ruined that plan.

Tommy thinks about his dad, wishes they could go fishing together, wishes his dad and mom got along better. He misses them, but not as much as he thought he would. Grandma told him he could call home tonight. He wants to be able to tell his mom and dad he caught a fish, a big one. He wants to tell them about the route they'll be taking, out to the Pacific Ocean tomorrow and then north along the coast towards Alaska. He'll tell them the highway numbers, the ones he's been memorizing from Grandpa's map. He wants them to be interested.

Tommy's thoughts shift to the older couple they met on the ferry three days ago. The couple kept referring to Tommy as Grandpa and Grandma's son. Grandpa corrected them the first time, but they kept on doing it, and Grandpa didn't stop them again. He had winked at Tommy and asked if he minded. Tommy said no, it was okay. For a second he felt guilty, as if he were betraying his dad, but he could tell Grandpa was pleased and, besides, he sometimes secretly wished that Grandpa were his dad.

Lucille takes her last mouthful of tea, puts down the plastic cup, and opens the thick book. She steals a quick glance at her boys, lets love of them wash over her, deliberately savoring the moment. She intends to use this memory later on, draw on it in harder times. She starts to read.

Doug isn't really listening to the story. Mostly he just likes to hear Lucille's voice rise and fall and to watch Tommy listening, curious to see what will catch his interest. It reminds him of his own mother reading. It only happened on Sundays. Other days she was too busy, had too many kids to run after. But on Sunday evenings she would gather them around, all 13 of them, and read. And something would change in her. Her face would soften, and Doug would feel a tenderness from her that he never felt at other times. He always hated going to bed on Sundays, always pressed her to read more, longer.

Doug is so pleased that he invited Tommy to join them on holiday. He's crazy about the kid, and the boy seems to be having a good time. Doug's always liked kids. He didn't mind being a surrogate parent to his younger siblings. And he was delirious when his own boys were born. It was only as they grew older that he started to push them too hard. If he could do it over, he'd be less concerned that they be the best at everything. He'd build them up instead of tearing them down.

Doug takes a deep breath, closes his eyes for a moment, feels the breeze on his face. So many mistakes he's made over the years. He's never really understood how he came to be so driven. Why was it so important to get ahead in the company? Why did he have to prove himself again and again to his family? Why did he push his boys relentlessly to succeed? Why did he turn bitter despite his achievements? It's no wonder he finally snapped, fell into a long and deep depression. It was terrible beyond words. But it's different now. He's not depressed and he hasn't felt driven the same way since he recovered from the depression.

Lucille reaches the end of a chapter, sticks the slip of paper in, and closes the book.

"I'm going to rest for a minute." She rummages through her bag looking for a lip balm. Finds it, rubs it across her lips. She notices Doug looking at her, smiles with her whole face. He smiles back. There were days when she thought she'd never see another smile like that from him. She's sure it's a miracle to feel this way again.

Doug is on her wavelength. He's thinking how good she looks and how grateful he is to her. Lucille stuck with him through the years of his depression and proved her love was deeper than he'd ever known. He's thankful he had the depression before being diagnosed with prostate cancer. Otherwise he knows he would be a basket case and making life miserable for Lucille. And while he's been doing pretty well, he still takes the antidepressants, just to be safe. He's learned from past experience that self-reliance has its limits. And he's also learned about what is really important in his life. Now even the impotence doesn't get him down, at least not very often. Every day he decides to be positive, decides not to be unhappy. It's hard work, but most days he's doing it.

"Hey!" It's Tommy, and his rod is bent sharply towards the water.

"I've got one!" He starts rotating the reel handle fiercely.

"Thattaboy! Bring him in." Lucille reaches over and pats him on the shoulder.

Doug can see that Tommy is too aggressive in playing the fish, worries that it will get away.

"Take your time, Tommy. Let him play himself out." Doug hears the critical edge to his voice, notices the desire to take the rod away from Tommy and do it properly.

He restrains the urge to step in, softens his tone. "You're doing just fine, son."

Tommy's face is alive. Joy one moment. Terror of losing the fish the next. The meaning of his life is landing this fish.

"Hand me the net, will you, Lucille?" Doug wants to be ready.

"There he is!" Tommy shouts as the trout breaks the surface of the lake about ten yards from the boat.

"Look how big he is."

"See if you can bring him up alongside here." Doug points, then lowers the net into the water.

The trout goes placid, and Tommy slowly reels him closer. Then it erupts into action, jerking this way and that. Tommy waits for the fight to ease, then reels him in next to the hull.

Doug brings the net up from underneath the trout, lifts it out of the water and then into the boat. Rainbow scales sparkle in the sun.

"I did it! I did it! Isn't he beautiful, Grandpa?"

"He's a real dandy. You did great!"

Tommy and Doug beam at each other.

Lucille is almost undone watching her ecstatic boys. Feeling silly, she dabs at her eyes with a tissue. And then, without warning, something changes. For the first time in ages, she knows that she can handle whatever the future may bring. Prostate cancer can't take this moment away. Nor can depression. She has enough inside her. Bring on the enemy. She and her boys are ready.

Prostate Cancer and Depression

Most men diagnosed with prostate cancer experience some symptoms of depression, at least intermittently. This is hardly surprising, given the many challenges involved with an illness experience. Indeed, individuals who learn of a cancer diagnosis, or of an illness recurrence, typically go through a series of reactions, including initial shock and disbelief, followed by mixed symptoms of anxiety and depression, irritability, and disruption of appetite and sleep. Concentration gets worse, and thoughts about cancer and the future intrude throughout the day and night. Over several weeks, the intensity of emotional turmoil usually lessens gradually, but may rise again as new medical crises develop.[1]

While it is helpful for men to know that initial emotional responses to prostate cancer are normal, it is also important not to minimize the impact of these responses. Writers about male depression argue that, for a variety of reasons, depression is a bigger problem than statistics show. Some men are depressed but express their struggles in other ways, such as through addictive behavior or aggression, and so never get identified as depressed.[2] Other men don't get diagnosed with depression because of health professional biases that result in under-diagnosis of men and over-diagnosis of women.[3] People with cancer are particularly likely not to have depression identified because symptoms get confounded with symptoms of the illness.[4]

While there is a continuum of depression that men may experience, those who experience the classic form of clinical depression show, for a duration of at least two weeks, signs of feeling sad, "down" and "blue," or having a decreased interest in pleasurable activities. In addition, men must exhibit at least four of the following symptoms: weight loss or gain, too little or too much sleep, fatigue, feelings of worthlessness or guilt, difficulty making decisions or forgetfulness, and preoccupation with death or suicide. Clinical depression is more likely for cancer patients with advanced disease.[1] While this may be related to concerns that ill people have about dying, it can also be related to physiological matters. When people are in pain, they're more likely to be depressed.[4] Depression is also a possible side effect of hormone treatments for prostate cancer,[5] and some research suggests that lower testosterone levels correlate with increased depression.[6]

Treatments for depression include a variety of medications (which are often very effective!), as well as psychological therapies.[1,4] Men experiencing depressive symptoms consistently for more than a few weeks should take action to get help. Once depression takes hold, it can be very difficult to shake, and individual will power is usually not sufficient to turn things around.

REFERENCES

1. Massie, M. J., & Popkin, M. K. (1998). Depressive disorders. In J.C. Holland (Ed.), *Psycho-oncology* (pp. 518-540). New York: Oxford University Press.

2. Real, T. (1997). *I don't want to talk about it*. New York: Fireside Books.

3. Potts, M. K., Burnam, M. A., & Wells, K. B. (1991). Gender differences in depression detection: A comparison of clinician diagnosis and standardized assessment. *Psychological Assessment, 3,* 609-615.

4. Spiegel, D. (1996). Cancer and depression. *British Journal of Psychiatry, 168,* 109-116.

5. Gleave, M. E., Bruchovsky, N., Moore, M. J., & Venner, P. (1999). Prostate cancer: Treatment of advanced disease. *Canadian Medical Association Journal, 160,* 225-232.

6. Steiger, A., von Bardeleben, U., Wiedemann, K., & Holsboer, F. (1991). Sleep EEG and nocturnal secretion of testosterone and cortisol in patients with major endogenous depression during acute phase and after remission. *Journal of Psychiatric Research, 25,* 169-177.

I Was Just a Number

The speaker is a 64-year-old white man who had a radical
prostatectomy 14 months ago and is currently disease free.
He is married and is an independent contractor.

I've always been in construction and on the move. It wasn't
unusual for me to work 12, 14, maybe 16 hours a day, seven days a
week. I mean, I don't want to brag, but I had this young fellow working with me, and he couldn't keep up with me. He'd be pooped and
have to rest when we got to the top of the stairs. But I just kept
going.

I had 63 years with no sickness. You get used to taking things
for granted. Like with your wife, you can have sex when it feels
right. And if you want to eat, you eat whatever you want. And you
get up and go to work and your body does what you want it to.

And then suddenly, you hit this brick wall, and you don't have
no control over anything anymore.

I was asking myself why this prostate cancer happened to me. I
didn't do nothing wrong. I didn't smoke. I was in good shape.
People looked at me, and they couldn't believe I was sick. I could-
n't believe it, either.

When I got home from the hospital, a nurse came and visited
me. I told her I didn't need her. I can change my own dressing. I said
I'm sure you could donate your time to somebody else. I'll take care
of myself. They gave me pills for pain. I read the side effects on the
bottle and went and threw them in the garbage. They want to relieve
you of one pain and give you another two. I didn't want that.

When we were kids in Bosnia we used to have rock-throwing fights. Once somebody got hurt, then we'd all run away, and the game was over. Then we'd do it over again the next day. Take my cousin, for example. You can't put your finger anywhere on his head without feeling scars from those rocks. When you got home, even if you were bleeding, you would never go and tell your mother. If you did, you'd just get a licking for getting into a fight. So you learned to keep your mouth shut and clean yourself up.

I had a few complications after the surgery. I went into kind of a depression. You know, you're used to a lifestyle, and suddenly you end up without your freedom. I mean, I understood that the recovery would be slow, but it was worse than I thought. I had no control over my peeing. If I would sneeze I would wet myself. And then I had an infection and they had to pump it out.

I went back to work too soon. I'd be okay for a couple of hours in the morning, but by 10 a.m. I wouldn't be able to lift a gallon of paint without wetting myself. So I tried to slow down, but I'm so used to pushing myself that I just got worse.

Where I grew up, in Bosnia, life was about survival. There was no room for lazy people. Everybody worked all the time. My mother bore 15 kids; four of us survived. There wasn't enough food. We slept in a barn. I've always felt it was important to work hard.

I kept working, and then I had a mild heart attack. My family doctor told me I had to slow down more, so I did. But it's been hard. I decided I had to quit getting into fights. I get pissed off so easily. You know, in my work I have to deal with engineers and architects, and sometimes they treat you like you're stupid because you don't have a university degree. And I would give them hell, wouldn't put up with their shit. But now I try not to get into it.

The sexual part isn't there anymore. All you can do is try and get used to that. We tried different methods, and as far as I'm concerned, there's nothing that can replace sex the way it was. Now with everything you have to do to have pleasure, it ends up not being pleasure at all. Sometimes it's a big urge, but what are you going to do?

You just lose morale. I mean, it's artificial, it's painful. It's just not a natural way anymore. It takes the desire away, and the fear comes in and then it doesn't work. Then you figure the hell with it. I mean, you just have to live without it.

I have to pull my penis and put the needle in it. And then it doesn't work. It burns, and I think, what am I doing to myself? So what kind of business is it that promotes this stuff? I mean, for five needles you pay a hundred bucks or whatever the hell it is. They can shove them up their ass. For all the good it did me.

At school, I finished grade four, and that was it. I had to go back and repeat it twice. The way it worked was that you had to leave so much food for the teacher in order to get moved on. We didn't have no food to give, so I did the same grade again. I would never have gotten past grade four.

I don't want to discuss sex. I just get upset, and then my blood pressure goes to hell. I'd like to close the subject and not deal with it anymore. I'm sorry, but that's just the way it is.

We went back to Bosnia this year. You see all that destruction, the houses all torn up, and the furniture full of bullet holes. You just get so upset. And it helped me to quit being depressed. I just thought, hey, what the hell do I have to complain about? So get off your bloody ass and get on with your life. I mean, I had to quit bellyaching and just try and be as happy as possible.

There's no sense crying over spilt milk.

But you should know that it wasn't my health that was the hardest to deal with. It was the way I got treated. I was working for a big company at the time I went for the surgery, and I was supposed to have medical coverage. Well, I did get covered for the period right after the surgery. But then, like I said, I went back to work too soon and was still wetting myself, and then I had a heart attack and was really depressed. I tried to get long-term disability coverage, but I couldn't. Around that time I went to see my family physician that I've had for 15 years. When she saw me she turned white as a sheet and dropped what she was doing. She said I looked like a dead person.

These insurance people, they didn't even see me. They didn't talk with me. Nothing. I'd leave a message, and no one would call me back. I went down there one time, and they said the person I wanted to see was unavailable. How do you know if they're telling the truth? I was just a number to them.

I went to talk with the people at the company, and they said it's not our fault, it's not our responsibility. And I said, well, that's a bunch of bullshit. Because you are the ones who selected this company to represent us in the first place, to protect us when we get sick. But, I mean, they just went on about all the benefits we get and blah, blah, blah. It just made me so pissed off. If I could ever find the person who made the decisions, I would spit in his face. Because I'm not trying to abuse the system. I'm just trying to get help when I need it. And they could care less.

They aren't interested in human beings. We're garbage to them. Just garbage.

I brought them my medical records to show that it was real. But they didn't even look at them. They just said I could go back to work. I told them to stick it up their ass and hired myself a lawyer. But I was getting too pissed off. I gave the lawyer two months to get a settlement, which he did, but all it did was pay his fees. But I knew I couldn't be waiting around forever for a proper deal because it would drive me crazy, and I'd probably have another heart attack. I'm sure they're happy now. They don't have to deal with me. They didn't want me getting sick on them again. They know how to screw the working person.

My neighbor across the street, her brother died of prostate cancer. He ended up in a wheelchair, and they kept sending this information. Threatening to cut him off disability unless he got all these forms filled out. Have you seen those bloody forms? What a bunch of bureaucratic bullshit. Now the doctors charge you to fill them out. And you're having to run around every few months and get these signatures. As if it wasn't obvious that this guy was dying. As if they thought he was running a little construction job on the side from his wheelchair. Bastards!

It's not good for me to talk too much about this. Before I got sick I'd never have let the bastards get away with treating me like garbage. But now I have to be careful. I had to let it go.

So I've been working for myself the past while. If everything goes well, I'm going to retire this year. But I'm not going to be sitting on my backside playing cards. I want to give back to society. We are part of society, and we have to support that. If there's any way to help I want to do it.

When we were in Bosnia, I went looking for the place where I grew up. It was terrible in a way, because when we were kids every square foot of land was used to grow something. Now it's virtually deserted. A wasteland. I found where our house used to be. I couldn't believe it. The walls of the house were still standing. But inside the walls and all around it had gone back entirely to nature. There was a big fig tree growing right in the middle of the house. It gave me goose bumps to see it. It gave me a kind of courage to go on.

WORK AND INSURANCE ISSUES

Most working people with cancer report that their jobs are helpful in sustaining a sense of emotional stability during difficult times.[1] Unfortunately (according to a large survey of U.S. cancer survivors, supervisors, and co-workers), cancer survivors are five times more likely to be laid off or fired than other workers. And they suffer from a wide variety of other discriminatory practices.[1] This occurs despite laws in the United States that prevent employers (prospective or existing) from treating cancer survivors differently from other employees. Loopholes exist, especially for smaller businesses, and so discriminatory practices are relatively common.

While many working people with cancer try to arrange treatment on a schedule that allows them to carry on with their jobs, this is not always possible. Men who choose surgery for prostate cancer, for example, need time to recuperate. Short-term disability benefits, usually lasting for a maximum of four to six months, are available for employees of some companies. Government-sponsored programs exist in both Canada and the United States to help employees without benefit plans with the means of taking necessary time off from work to recover from treatment.[1,2] Finding out about these programs, and successfully completing the application process, is not always straightforward.

Men who have long-term disability benefit plans available through their workplace are even more likely to have difficulty claiming benefits. Medical forms must be submitted after short-term benefits are exhausted, sometimes by all treating physicians and specialists, and the case must be made that the individual is totally incapable of doing his former job. Later, the case must be made that he is unable to do any job offered by the company. Physicians typically charge for reports. For men initially approved for coverage, updates must be provided every few months. While the frequency of reports may lessen over time for men who remain ill, there is no guarantee of this, and insurance companies are likely to request that patients undergo periodic examinations by their doctors and/or work assessments.

In the United States, health insurance policies are usually accessed through private employers or insurance companies. Once an individual has been diagnosed with cancer, especially for the first couple of years, it becomes much more difficult to purchase private health insurance plans. If applications are eventually accepted, substantially higher premiums are a certainty.

The U.S. government provides insurance to selected individuals based on age, income, and/or health status. In Canada, government-provided health insurance is available to all. But health insurance plans (privately and publicly funded) vary greatly, so that services provided under one plan may not be provided under another. This is especially so for services that may not be deemed necessary—

*experimental drugs, rehabilitation services such as physio-
therapy and complementary approaches like naturopathy.
Also, access to services changes over time. For example,
access to a range of publicly funded services in Canada is
declining, leading more people to purchase "extended
health insurance" plans.*

REFERENCES

1. Canadian Breast Cancer Network. (2001). Extended health
benefits for breast cancer survivors. Available at www.cbcn.ca.
2. Hoffman, B. (2001). *Working it out: Your employment rights
as a cancer survivor* (5th edition). Washington, DC: National
Coalition for Cancer Survivorship.

Simon Cultivates Romance

*Simon is a 63-year-old white man who was diag-
nosed eight years ago. He originally had surgery,
then radiation therapy, and now is on long-term
hormone therapy. He has also tried many alternative treatments. He is married to a younger woman
and recently sold his property management business.*

Simon scrolls down the list on his computer screen. Day excur-
sions from Bangkok. He likes the look of the one that includes a stop
at an ancient Buddhist monastery in the Thai forest. Monasteries
have always intrigued him.

The knock startles him. He swivels the chair towards the door,
finds himself face to face with a midriff. He leans forward and kisses
its flat surface, then looks up, past the breasts he knows and loves,
meets Lynda's clear blue eyes. He takes in the wide smiling mouth,
the loose strands of wavy blond hair. What a fine looking woman.

"How're you doing, lover?" She reaches out a hand and strokes
the side of his head.

"Great. I was just checking out tour possibilities for if we decide
to go ahead and do that Thailand trip next spring."

"I hope we can do it." The look on her face is one part hope, one
part worry.

"I don't see why not. The money isn't a problem. And with any
luck the hormone treatment will keep the cancer at bay." He hears the
strained edge to his voice, the optimism harder to count on these days.

"Let's plan for it. But first we have the Florida trip. Have you made arrangements yet?"

"I was going to head over to the travel agent in a few minutes to do just that. Want to come?"

"No. Marilyn's on her way over to pick me up. She wants to do some shopping, maybe go and look at that new furniture store we saw over on Shepphard Avenue. I won't be late. You remember, don't you, that we're having a special dinner tonight?"

"You bet I do." He grabs her hand and squeezes.

"And it won't be just the dinner that's special." She leans over and gives him the total blue eye look, kisses him hard on the lips.

"Every moment with you is special." He means it. And he's determined that it will be special tonight, that he'll come through for her. He won't allow another disaster.

The doorbell rings and then Lynda's gone. Simon shuts down the computer. Then he feels the hot flash coming on, sits back down and rides it through, waving a magazine in front of his face. When it finally ends, he sighs deeply, makes the effort to sidestep discouragement. He decides to drop off some documents at his former business on the way to the travel agent and goes looking for them in a filing cabinet. Officially, he's been retired since the cancer came back, but the new owners keep finding reasons to ask for his help. He complains about it to Lynda, but the truth is he likes being useful. After all those years hustling to build the business, it's hard to just walk away. And he'd hate to see his success not continue under the new owners.

He heads out, documents in hand. Notices that the lawn needs cutting and reminds himself to phone the guy who's supposed to be doing it. It galls him not to have the energy to do all the upkeep anymore. And he hates the thought of moving to a smaller place, was angry with Lynda when she brought it up last week. Told her to quit being so negative about his health. Immediately apologized, and so he should have. Nobody could be more positive, more supportive than Lynda has been.

They were only a year into the marriage when he was diagnosed with the prostate cancer. He told her to leave then, that it had been a mistake for her to marry an older man. She told him to forget that nonsense, that she was with him come hell or high water. She'd had some of both in the last eight years. He doesn't know what he would have done without her. He owes her big time. He wants to do everything he can to be there for her.

At the office, he chats for a few minutes with his secretary. She worked for him for 20 years, knows him in some ways better than Lynda or, for that matter, his ex-wife, Marty. He misses the office routines, misses being around her. And he can tell she misses him, too.

At the travel agent, he goes over all the details. Everyone is coming and going at the beach house on different schedules. His daughter and her family are coming early and leaving early so his son-in-law can get to a big business meeting in New Orleans. His son and daughter-in-law are coming later, after classes end and he finishes marking report cards. Simon and Lynda will go a week before everyone else. Time to be alone together. Time to walk on the beach, to take it easy, to cultivate romance. Everything will go on his credit card. What's the point in making all that money if you don't spend it on the people who count? And maybe it partly makes up for his neglect of the kids while they were growing up.

He says goodbye to the agent, drives to the pharmacy to pick up his prescription and syringes. The thought of the injections doesn't scare him anymore. Now the fear is all about whether the drugs will do the job. Whether they will get his penis hard and whether they will keep it hard. He's not sure. That's why they've decided to add the vacuum pump to the injections this time. He doesn't like the pump and hasn't used it in a long time. But whatever it takes. Lynda's such a sensuous woman. She needs him. He's determined for it to work.

Standing in line at the cash register, he re-reads the pamphlet about side effects. "Penile pain/ache." Yeah, well, that's about what you could expect from sticking a needle into the shaft of your penis. "Prolonged erection." He doesn't even want to think about that one, about the night he had to sit for hours in the Emergency with the world's most painful hard-on. Talk about tough. The fiddling with dosages seemed to go on forever before they finally got it right. But the injections weren't even the starting place; they came only after other disappointments. Like the Viagra adventure that only managed to give him an enormous headache. And the vacuum pump that took forever to figure out and then broke the second time they used it. It's only recently that the replacement parts came in. And then there were the various herbal concoctions, a total waste of time.

It's been a struggle since the surgery. The surgeon preserved the nerves on one side but had to cut the ones on the other side. He said that the best Simon could expect would be partial erections. So as soon as he'd recovered from the surgery, Simon started experimenting with aids. Mostly, they found ways to keep their sex life on track. And even when the technologies didn't do the trick, they stayed positive, stayed turned on, fuelled by their mutual desires. But that was then and this is now. Things are different.

Simon hands over his money to the cashier. He resists rubbing his nipples until he gets to the car. He can't believe how much they hurt, wishes he'd worn a softer shirt, wishes he didn't have to take the hormones that cause the hot flashes and make his breasts so big and sore. It's time to head home. Time to get himself ready for tonight. It's just been so much harder since he started the hormone treatments. When they first told him the cancer had spread, he refused the hormones. Went crazy with vitamins. Tried acupuncture. Ingested turmeric and soy protein. Got serious about his diet. But his PSA readings kept going up, and he finally gave in and started on a combined hormone blockade of testosterone. PSA readings started going down. And, predictably, Simon lost his desire for sex. These days, he's about as interested in sex as he is in a box of tissue.

He hates his apathy about sex, tries to manufacture desire, and pretends to Lynda that he feels it. He's frantic to find ways to carry on with lovemaking. But it hasn't been going very well. At the last visit to his urologist, they had him fill out those stupid quality-of-life scales again. On a scale of one to ten, where one is really great and ten is incredibly awful, how is your sex life? He marked himself at eight, but is trying like hell to get back to seven.

Back at home, he's not surprised that Lynda's not there. Simon phones the yard maintenance guy, leaves a message that he wants the lawn cut tomorrow or else. Then he gets the vacuum pump out of his dresser drawer, reminds himself how it works.

He decides to try and get a jump-start on arousal. Takes himself to the entertainment room in the basement, starts combing through the film library. His eye catches on one with Lynda's handwriting, "Love in Florida." It's a home-made film, one of several experiments in documenting their lovemaking. This one was taken a few months after their marriage, and he hasn't watched it for at least a couple of years.

He presses play, and images appear on the five-foot screen. His first impression is of how much younger they both look, especially him. Then he is struck by the playful ease with which they embrace and undress each other. He detects no awkwardness between them. These familiar actors seem entirely absorbed with each other, oblivious to the camera, oblivious to the possibility that their lovemaking could ever be anything but wonderful. It hurts to watch them making love. He aches for that time, for the easy abandon they once had with each other. He presses the stop button.

He shakes his head to try and clear the images of his former self. He searches through the library for something else, something less personal. He finds an erotic film that they bought at the nearby sex shop. It features a slow seduction scene at a restaurant. A man and a woman are making conversation with others at their table, trying to interact normally with a waiter—and all the time engaging in a tentative, then insistent, under-the-table interaction. The film used to turn him on, but now he watches with detached curiosity. Mentally, he senses a kind of titillation. It borders on desire, but isn't quite desire. He tries to find his way into full-blown desire, tries to will his mind to override his dormant body. He imagines himself in the restaurant with that gorgeous long-legged redhead. He strokes himself. He stops. Shuts off the machines. Kicks the sofa. Walks slowly upstairs. Lies down on their bed. Sleeps.

He wakes to the sound of Spanish guitar and the spiced scent of his favorite chicken dish. He smiles to himself, knowing that the dance has begun. He feels a fierce rush of love for Lynda. Slides into his slippers and goes to find her, telling himself just to focus on her, telling himself that everything will be okay.

Lynda is wearing a new loose-fitting blouse, swirls of various shades of green, and a new cream-colored skirt. She tells him she bought them today on sale. He admires how she looks, which is easy to do. Doesn't say anything about her spending habits, not even when she tells him about the new dining room table that Marilyn encouraged her to order. He reminds himself that he should be pleased to give what he can.

Dinner proceeds at a leisurely pace. A glass of wine. Lynda repeats the stories about mutual friends that she's heard from Marilyn. Tossed salad. Simon tells her the news from his secretary, about the former employee who landed in jail. Tomato basil soup from the local gourmet shop. They chat about the Florida trip, places they want to go for dinner, people they'd like to see. Chicken and roast potatoes and carrots. They reminisce. Lynda tells the story again, the one about the first time she met him, about how she knew he was the one. He jokes with her in the familiar way. Makes himself out as an innocent, drawn in by the wiles of a beautiful woman.

They move to sit in the solarium and watch the sun setting over the back hedge, speaking quietly and then not at all. Her fingers lightly stroke the inside of his forearm. His hand rests gently on the back of her neck. With the sun's red finally gone, she takes his hand and leads him inside. The syringe waits for them on the bedside table. Lynda takes charge. He is grateful that she does.

"Lean back, darling. This will just take a second. Do you remember that beach in Costa Rica? The time we made love under the stars?"

He closes his eyes. Pictures of the beach take shape, but he can't hold onto them. He's all too aware of her hand on the head of his penis, pulling it taut to smooth out the skin. He knows she's lining up the needle. The injection will be at the ten o'clock position, about a third of the way up the shaft. They used the two o'clock position last time. He feels the cold steel against his skin.

"Do you remember the outfit I was wearing that night?"

She's trying to distract him. It partly works. He remembers the halter top, can almost taste the ocean salt on her lips.

"Augh!" The needle is in, thank God. He holds his breath, waits for the syringe to empty into him. Lynda carefully extracts the needle, grabs a piece of cotton batting and presses against the injection site. He takes it from her, has a look. Not too much blood. He hopes there won't be so much bruising this time.

"Keep pressing, love." Her voice is soft. She leans over and kisses the corner of his mouth. He holds the cotton tight to his penis. He watches as she stands and slowly removes pieces of clothing. They sit naked on the bed, waiting.

He looks into her eyes. He sees unwept tears. He sees tender love for him. He sees her pained desire.

She looks into his eyes. She sees his fear. She sees his hope. She sees the man she married, the one who won her heart. She sees his devotion to her.

They touch. They stroke slowly. They kiss. His penis starts to grow. They smile at the same moment.

He pulls out the vacuum pump from the drawer, fits the cylinder over his penis. He starts the pump and a vacuum is created around his penis, triggering blood to flow in. The erection is growing. Lynda arranges the tension band at the base of the penis, designed to keep it upright after the cylinder is removed.

They proudly survey their handiwork. One erect penis.

Lynda wants him to enter her right away, not wanting to miss the opportunity while it's there. She's suddenly feeling how much she's been missing him.

Inside her, Simon initially moves slowly, then quickens his pace. He narrows his attention to the sensation in his penis, to Lynda's low moans, to the bite of her nails in the small of his back. He feels the pressure growing inside him, the hope of release. Pushes harder, faster, wanting to get there. Lynda rises to meet him, louder now. But he doesn't come, seems stuck on a plateau. Loses his focus.

A thought: "Maybe it isn't going to work."

A counter-thought: "Don't give up. You love this woman."

A thought: "Is it getting softer?"

A counter-thought: "Stay focused. Remember the beach on Costa Rica."

A thought: "Shit, I'm losing it. God, help me!"

Another thought: "I can't fail again. I just can't."

Another thought: "I love this woman. But I'm no good to her."

They lie together in silence. He's on his back staring at the ceiling. She has one leg draped across him, head lying on his shoulder. They both tried to save things. She encouraged other positions, took him in her mouth. Later, after it was clear he couldn't respond, he offered to bring her to climax. She said no, she'd rather wait and try again another time. Maybe on the weekend.

He desperately searches inside himself for some glint of hope, some place of consolation. He says things to himself. Maybe it will be better next time. If he just tries harder. At least they love each other, can show their love in other ways.

Positive thinking just doesn't cut it. Desolation wells up. A wave of despair grows. Bigger.

The wave crashes against rocks. Tears stream down his face, and his body convulses. A different kind of release. Lynda holds him tight, makes soothing sounds, strokes his face. A different kind of intimacy. Childlike. Letting himself be taken care of, letting himself be totally vulnerable. He feels his love, feels his deep debt to her. He sleeps.

Later, in the dark of the night, he is awake, his brief illusion of peace long gone. What can he do? Maybe he should run away, live out his end days with a bottle. But he knows he can't, that it would be even worse for Lynda. Maybe it's time to get a permanent prosthesis to keep his penis erect. He hasn't wanted to do it because it's the last step, irreversible. It means admitting to himself that things will never get better, admitting that there will never be another starlit night on a beach in Costa Rica.

He feels the tears begin to well again, forces them back with an act of will. He'll make an appointment with the urologist tomorrow. Maybe he can get the procedure done before they go to Florida. He's going to make sure they have the best vacation ever.

METASTATIC DISEASE AND HORMONE TREATMENTS

When cancer has metastasized (i.e., spread beyond the region of the prostate), it is no longer curable. However, when treatment is instigated to alter the levels of testosterone and other male sex hormones, the disease can be kept from progressing for a number of years, allowing men to live longer.[1] Treatment is aimed to produce very low levels of testosterone, called "castrate levels." This is achieved either through surgical removal of the testicles or through various drug regimens. Many men are understandably reluctant to select the surgical option.

One major impact of reducing male hormone levels is a dramatic loss of interest in sex, along with an overall lessening of energy. For many men, these are saddening developments, challenging to adjust to. The capacity for erections is increasingly compromised the longer that men stay on drugs. Hot flashes are another side effect, although medication can usually help control them. Over time, the male body undergoes feminizing changes: muscle mass diminishes, and the body takes on a somewhat rounder shape. Breast enlargement and sensitivity occurs with some drug treatments. Osteoporosis frequently develops.[2]

The impact on men of radical changes in hormone levels has received insufficient research attention. It is especially important to better understand how some men carry on active, full lives for many years while simultaneously dealing with substantial treatment effects.

REFERENCES

1. Gleave, M. E., Bruchovsky, N., Moore, M. J., & Venner, P. (1999). Prostate cancer: Treatment of advanced disease. *Canadian Medical Association Journal, 160*, 225-232.

2. Klotz, L. (2000). *Prostate cancer: A guide for patients.* Toronto: Prospero Books.

Darren Celebrates a Birthday

Darren is a 60-year-old white gay man who was diagnosed seven years ago. He has had radiation therapy and hormone therapy, but now is being treated with experimental chemotherapy. Pain control is an issue. He has a long-term partner and is not able to work.

Darren closes his eyes, just for a few seconds, not wanting to doze off again. When he opens them, Vlad is sitting quietly by his bedside, absorbed in reading. Darren reaches out with his right hand, the one without the I.V. tube attached, touches Vlad's knee. Their eyes meet.

"You should have woken me." Darren hates to miss any of the time they have together. Especially this morning, when he has things he wants to say.

"I couldn't bear to do it. You looked so peaceful." Tears well in Vlad's eyes. "I'm just so glad that you're able to sleep now. It was awful to see you in pain like that."

Darren feels his own tears forming, partly shared relief from his recent ordeal, partly his tenderness for Vlad. He worries about how tired Vlad looks, about the cost of his illness for his partner. That's what he wants to talk about.

Vlad is digging in his cotton shopping bag, pulls out a small, brightly wrapped package, bowed and ribboned. "Happy birthday, lover." He leans over and kisses Darren lightly on the lips. Darren savors the kiss, marveling at the intimacy that long ago went beyond passion, becoming something more exquisite, sublime even. And more painful.

"There's a bigger present waiting for you when you get home. I talked to the doctor last night, and he said you should be able to leave in another day or so."

"Thanks, Vlad." Darren can't stop smiling. He's delighted about the possibility of going home. Delighted about being almost entirely pain-free. Delighted that he's still here for his sixtieth birthday. He thinks that he's a very lucky man. But he does have something on his mind.

"I've been wanting to talk with you." Darren can hear that his speech is slow, his voice weaker than it used to be. But he really wants to say this. He's had too much experience with friends with AIDS to be able to deny the effect of his prostate cancer on Vlad. He refuses to let himself assume that things can continue as they have. So many times he's seen it, how partners hit a point where they simply can't give any more, can't continue to bear the burden, have to abandon the ill person for their own survival. It's not that Vlad has given any indication of wanting to leave, but Darren knows he must want to at times. Or at least he imagines so. Vlad has been a wonderful support from the beginning. Darren was surprised at how eagerly he took up the challenge, was surprised at how their relationship took a deeper turn, how their love bloomed in new ways. But it's been a lot of years since the diagnosis. And now that the cancer has spread through his bones ....

"You know things haven't been going so well lately. And they're not going to get any better. I see you come here in the morning looking worried and tired, and then you go off to that horrible job all day, and then you're back here in the evening looking even more worn out. I never wanted this for you."

Vlad is scratching his head fiercely, looking agitated. Darren puts up his hand, palm outwards. "Just let me finish."

Vlad stops scratching.

"I want you to think about your options. I'm not expecting you to keep taking care of me. You've already done more than I could have asked ...."

"Okay, that's enough, Darren." Vlad's voice has an angry edge to it. "I know what my options are, and I'm choosing to be with you and ...."

He stops mid-sentence, leans closer, "I love you, and you're stuck with me." He leans back again. "So quit misbehaving, and enjoy your birthday."

Darren gives in happily. He wants Vlad in his life, no doubt about it. He's feeling again how lucky he is.

Vlad gets to his feet. "Listen, I've got to go. I can't afford to keep the dragon lady waiting again. We have a meeting at nine to go over the budget."

"Don't let her abuse you." Darren says it jokingly, but he wishes Vlad had a more sympathetic boss.

Vlad kisses the top of Darren's bald head, hair loss being the only noticeable impact so far of the new chemotherapy regime.

"See you tonight."

"Bye, Vlad."

Darren is suddenly tired. He thinks he'll close his eyes, but only for a second.

He opens his eyes, sensing a presence in the room. April is standing there, beaming down at him. He beams back, pleased as always to see her. She takes his hand, kisses the palm gently.

"How're you doing today, Darren?"

"Better, thanks. What time is it?"

"Just after ten."

"Wow. I must have slept for two hours."

"You must have needed it. I can't stay long, but I wanted to drop in and say happy birthday. You know you're one of the special people in my life, but I wanted you to hear it from my lips."

He's on the verge of tears again. He wonders if it's the medication that's making him weepy. Or whether, now that his time is running out, it's easier to be in touch with his feelings. He can't get over how grateful he's been feeling lately, not depressed like he'd anticipated.

"You and me, we go back a long ways …." He can't keep going. Tears are rolling down his cheeks. He moves to wipe them away.

April sits, pats his hand as if he were a troubled child.

"We sure do. And I don't regret any of it."

The tears keep flowing, resisting Darren's will to stop them. All they've been through together overwhelms him. The dissolving of their marriage when he finally came out publicly as a gay man. The working to maintain a sense of family, to make things okay for the kids. The constant reaching out to each other across the pain, managing to stay in love despite it all. A different kind of love, for sure, but still something quite wonderful.

"Thanks for everything, April." It doesn't seem enough; it seems there should be something more that could be said that would make it up to her.

April puts a finger on his lips. "I love you, Darren … and I hope you get out of here soon. I have a message from Val. She said she wanted to come this morning, but she has to hand in a paper tomorrow and needed to keep working on it. She'll come tonight."

Darren smiles to himself, thinking of his feisty youngest daughter, looking forward to seeing her. In another part of his mind, he's hoping she doesn't arrive at the same time as Vlad. They're polite to each other, but that's as good as it gets. Darren has learned the hard way that he can't make everyone into the best of friends.

April continues, "She'll bring our gift. So you'll just have to be patient."

"If I have to."

They share a smile that seems to go on and on, somehow including everything they've shared together over the years. He likes this woman immensely.

April is back on her feet. "Bye now. I'll call you tomorrow."

"Bye, April."

Darren dozes. When he wakes, he's alone. Sunlight streams through the window, covering most of his bed. For some reason he's entranced by this sun, soaks in it, would swim in it if he could. He's unaccountably delighted by the dust particles dancing in the light, watches them for a long time. When he looks out the window, he's startled by the sparkles on the nearby pond, wonders why he's never quite seen it this way before, so incredibly beautiful. His attention moves to tree branches, to the way they exquisitely thrust themselves into the blue of sky. And then he finds the clouds, rolling their whiteness out like ballet in slow motion. He feels like he could watch them all day and not tire of it. He rests in their graceful rhythms. And he's sure he's never been so happy.

The knock on the door startles him. It's Tracy, one of the nurses.

"It seems like they forgot to send you a lunch tray today. So we'll phone down to the kitchen and ask them to make up a sandwich or something. But it's hard to say if they'll get anything for you, they're so busy down there." She sounds harried, impatient.

"Oh ... I'd appreciate your trying. I'm kind of hungry." And suddenly he is hungry, incredibly hungry.

"Can't promise anything." And she's gone.

Darren is surprised by the interaction. The nurses and aids have all been so incredibly supportive in recent days. He's felt that they've taken a special interest in him, have taken good care of him. It's been unusual to get this kind of offhand treatment. And now he can't help feeling a bit sorry for himself about having no food, especially being his birthday and all. He decides he'll ring the nursing station again in another half an hour if nothing arrives by then.

He's no sooner turned to look out the window before there's another knock on the door.

Tracy walks in, smiling this time. After Tracy there are other nurses, and members of the cleaning staff and the food services staff. The last one has a lunch tray, and then after her, Val, his daughter, walks in carrying a cupcake with a candle stuck in it. And they all start singing "Happy Birthday to You."

Darren loses it, tears once again flowing freely down his face. This time, it doesn't bother him. Doesn't bother him a bit. He's just thinking what a lucky man he is. What a lucky man!

HORMONE REFRACTORY DISEASE AND PALLIATIVE CARE

Eventually, hormone treatments lose their power to control the spread of cancer. When men reach this point, they are faced with a situation where there are no proven strategies for extending life span.[1] Some men will try chemotherapy or other experimental medical approaches. Others will consider complementary/alternative approaches (e.g., naturopathy, homeopathy)—although studies have shown that many men are trying these approaches well before they're dealing with advanced disease.[2] Still other men will choose to stop treatments focused on the effort to lengthen their lives.

Whatever the choices men with hormone refractory prostate cancer make about trying to extend their lives, they and their doctors typically face more issues around quality of life. Controlling symptoms becomes an important priority. Bone pain becomes problematic for many, so it's important for men to seek medical assistance if this occurs. There have been important advances in pain control techniques in the last couple of decades; ill people deserve to benefit from these advances. Unfortunately, many men, and some health professionals, worry about the possible addictive effects of pain medications. This concern is not relevant for people with cancer. Aside from analgesics, radiation treatment and chemotherapy both can be useful in helping alleviate pain.[3]

It is clear that quality of life for men with advanced cancer is heavily influenced by good symptom control and expert attention from health care professionals. But this is not the whole story. Support from family and close friends makes a difference. And the meaning that men make of their lives, both past and present, affects how they experience their final months.[4]

REFERENCES

1. Klotz, L. (2000). *Prostate cancer: A guide for patients.* Toronto: Prospero Books.

2. Gray, R. E., Greenberg, M., Fitch, M., Parry, N., Douglas, M. S., & Labrecque, M. (1997). Perspectives of cancer survivors interested in unconventional cancer therapies. *Journal of Psychosocial Oncology, 15*, 49-71.

3. Iscoe, N. A., Bruera, E., & Choo, R. (1999). Prostate cancer: Palliative care. *Canadian Medical Association Journal, 160*, 365-371.

4. Lewis, F. M. (1989). Attributions of control, experienced meaning, and psychosocial well-being in patients with advanced cancer. *Journal of Psychosocial Oncology, 7*, 105-119.

No Big Deal?

By Vrenia Ivonoffski and Ross Gray

BATTLE SCENE

A man and a woman, wearing army helmets, come to center stage. The sound of bombs and machine gun fire is heard in the background.

Man 1: So this is it. Time to go into battle.

Woman 1: I guess there's nothing for us but to do our best.

Man 1: Yeah, we'll do what we need to do. Keep the casualties to a minimum.

Woman 1: It won't be so bad. We're a good fighting team.

Man 1: You're right. It will be over in no time, and we'll look back and laugh about this. (*A large bomb goes off, and the couple flee upstage.*)

Woman 1: (*Shouting as she runs.*) All we have to do is stay positive.

PROLOGUE

Man 2:   This presentation is about men facing illness. It's also about the women in their lives. The presentation is based on a study conducted by a research team at the Toronto Sunnybrook Regional Cancer Center and funded by the Canadian Cancer Society. Thirty-four men diagnosed with prostate cancer were each interviewed three times—before they had surgery to remove their prostate, two months after surgery, and a year later. Their spouses were also interviewed at each of these points in time. Most of the voices you will hear in this presentation are drawn directly from interview transcripts....

VENUS AND MARS

Man 3 (Professor Joker): (*Rushing forward and interrupting Man 2.*) Excuse me. Sorry I'm late. This is the prostate cancer forum? Right? (*Appeals to audience, then turns to Man 2.*) Thanks very much for holding down the fort. You can go now. (*Man 2 exits.*) As you all know, I'm Professor Joker. (*Encourages audience to clap.*)

Now, the first point I wish to make is that when a man gets sick it's a challenge for the space program. As you are all aware, and I must say that my own work has been critical to this matter, science has now firmly established that women are from Venus and men are from Mars. Those of you in a relationship know that communication between men and women can be a tad trying at the best of times. Throw in a man who is ill, and it's suddenly more like men and women are from different universes. So scientists need to be working on ways for men and women to travel back and forth across these huge distances.

The saving grace is that we're talking about men here. I mean, if it were women who were ill, well, then we'd have to worry about serious distress, you know, weeping and wailing and that kind of thing. But my research into the emotional lives of men shows that men are more similar to slabs of granite than they are to women. There's this ridiculous idea, promoted by a group of female scientists in the U.S., that men are just repressing stuff like fear of death, grief about aging, and so on, but my team is on the verge of proving, once and for all, that for men, it's really all NO BIG DEAL! (*Exits.*)

CROSS-DRESSING SCENE

Man 1 and Man 2, dressed in women's hats, come to center stage as female characters, carrying shopping bags. Man 3, also dressed as a woman, joins later.

Man 2:   Hi, Miriam. Thanks so much for the coffee cake recipe. Jack loved it.

Man 1:   Great. How is Jack?

Man 2:   Don't ask. He seems to be coming down with something, and so he's in one of his, "I'm fine, don't talk to me" moods.

Man 1:   Men! As soon as there's anything wrong, they clam up.

Man 2:   Let's face it. We women can talk about our bodies.

After periods, babies, and menopause, there's nothing sacred any more.

Man 1:   I guess that's helped us to cope—complain, share, get advice. But men have been taught to hold it all in.

Man 3:   Can you imagine a guy sitting around with his buddies, saying, "I have this pain in the family jewels. Do you ever have that?" (*Men all laugh.*)

Man 2:   Not likely.

Man 2 removes his wig and steps forward. Men 1 and 3 exit.

Man 2 (Jack):

Men are the strong, dominant type, sitting on horseback leading the troops. I know I'm not supposed to say that. But I can't get away from my background, my upbringing. I try not to be like that, but it's still there. And to a certain extent, I believe it's true.

PROFESSOR JOKER ON THE DIGITAL RECTAL EXAM

Man 3 (Professor Joker):

Greetings! Today I have extremely important information for you about prostates, direct from the front lines of medical science. I won't waste your precious time describing the prostate gland. I mean, Canadian men already know that prostates are about the size of a walnut and are located below their bladders. Right?! And everybody knows that prostate cancer is the most common type of cancer among men and that you have to be on the lookout for it. So let's not dwell on irrelevancies. Let's get on with the exciting news.

Isn't science wonderful, always moving from one frontier to the next? I'd like to draw your attention to an amazing medical intervention. You've heard of the precise technologies of the MRI and of laser surgery.

Now we have the DIGITAL RECTAL EXAM. This examination requires a highly adaptable instrument, the digit (*holding up finger*), which is employed by brave-hearted physicians to assess a man's prostate for abnormalities. The scientific term for these abnormalities, which I don't expect you to remember, is "bumps." The complex intervention involves the physician inserting the digit into a bodily cavity of the nether regions and feeling for bumps (*mime inserting, moving around in circles*). Of course, finding a bump may or may not mean there's a real problem, but you'll get to go through all kinds of other fascinating tests to find out for sure.

The digital rectal exam is, of course, easy, painless and altogether *No Big Deal*. Science has clearly revealed this to be true. My team surveyed 1,000 men that received digital rectal exams. Of the 17 who returned the survey, only four scrawled profanities across the page, leading us to conclude that most men don't mind the digital rectal exam in the least.

Training of doctors to conduct the digital rectal exam is extensive, requiring hundreds of hours of intensive application. So, men, don't try this at home! Here's the message to remember. Be responsible citizens, catch the wave, and celebrate medical science. Get your digital rectal exam today! (*Exits.*)

Woman 2 (Susan):

(*Coming forward to stand next to Jack.*) Jack and I have been married for 26 years. We are each other's best friends. And now, in my 50s I've had to think about what it would be like to be a widow. That's a wake-up call! Jack's been diagnosed with prostate cancer. I know cancer is a bad word, but, to tell you the truth, I was relieved it wasn't some other cancer. Prostate's the safe cancer, right? Wrong. I didn't know men could die of prostate cancer until we started reading about it. But you don't want to dwell on that. There are enough other worries even if they manage to get rid of the cancer—like impotence or incontinence or both. Jack gets annoyed and says, "We'll deal with it if and when it happens." So I back off. But if we're looking at the possibility of no more normal sex life, shouldn't we be discussing that? Shouldn't we be preparing ourselves? I know sex is really important to him. He must be more anxious than he's letting on. (*Jack and Susan exit.*)

FRED AND MIRIAM

Man 1 (Fred):

I've always thought men were more stoic than women, the ones I know anyway. They take things in their stride. I was raised in Cochrane, which is a mining town, and many years ago I was in the hospital. There were several guys in the room, and they had cancer and knew they were dying. They were laughing and joking. I thought they faced it all very well.

Woman 1 (Miriam):

My Fred is a good man—solid, dependable, hard-working. A man's man. He's not one to make a fuss when things go wrong, especially with his health. Now it seems he might have prostate problems, and my stomach's been in a knot ever since we found out he'll need tests. Fred seems to be able to put the whole thing aside while we wait and carry on as normal. I'm trying to do the same, for his sake, but it's so hard. I'll be so glad when we know something for sure. (*Fred and Miriam exit.*)

Man 3: I'm not so tough as I was. I'm tough mentally. I'm not as tough physically and emotionally. And that's kind of hard to deal with because you feel you're letting the side down. (*Exits.*)

Man 2: (*Coming to center stage with hockey stick.*) Waiting for a diagnosis is like a face-off in hockey: there's a lot of tension waiting for the puck to drop.

PROFESSOR JOKER ON PSA TESTS

Man 3 (Professor Joker):

(*Speaking rapidly, waving arms.*) Remember P.S.A.? The Prostate Specific Antigen? Well, here's what you need to know about PSA blood testing. It can help identify prostate cancers, but there's not a lot of evidence that our treatments of prostate cancer help in many cases. You might be better off not knowing. You might have prostate cancer, but you may end up dying of something else anyway. And if you have treatment, then you might end up with E.D.—erectile dysfunction—and maybe you'll be incontinent, and maybe none of it was really necessary. And though you might have a high PSA, it may not turn out to be prostate cancer. So you go through getting all upset for no good reason. But if it turns out you have prostate cancer and have a high Gleason score, then you'll probably be glad you had the test because you might have a chance to cure it. But if it's in an advanced stage, then you'll be kicking yourself that you didn't have it earlier.

Any questions? See me in my office. (*Exits.*)

DISORIENTATION—BATTLE SCENE

Woman 1: (*Holding map and frantically turning it around.*) Where are we? This map is useless. I can't even tell which side is up. And the roads aren't marked.

Man 1: (*Stumbling on stage breathless.*) Captain, the radar's not working, and we don't have any ammunition.

Woman 1: Well, how are we supposed to fight when we're not even sure where we are, where the enemy is, and what we're fighting with? (*Soldiers exit.*)

Man 2: (*Carrying hockey stick.*) Going to the doctor is like hockey. You never know when you're going to be blindsided by a body check.

HOSPITAL SCENE

Background hospital loudspeaker announcements—"Doctor Klein, Doctor Klein, please come to B-West nursing station."

Woman 1 (Miriam) is on the phone to her son. She and Fred are in a hospital room. Fred is folding his dressing gown, but making a mess of it.

Miriam: (*Speaking into phone.*) It's taken us four months to get in here, and now the doctor finally shows up after three days and tells us Dad has to leave because they need the bed. And he hadn't even looked at the biopsy results. Can you believe it? We asked him to go look at them before we leave. I'm so angry I could just spit bullets.

Fred: Simmer down, Miriam. They need the bed.

Miriam: And your Dad is being so agreeable about it all.

Fred: There's nothing we can do about it. Stop fussing.

Miriam: Oh Fred! (*Miriam grabs the dressing gown from Fred to fold it properly.*) I'll keep you posted, son. Bye. (*Doctor appears at the door.*) Doctor … what did you find out?

Man 3 (Doctor):
(*Standing in the doorway.*) Well, there's cancer there. I've left two prescriptions on the counter. You might want to read up on it. Come and see me in my office in six weeks, and we'll discuss your options. (*Exits.*)

(*Fred and Miriam look at each other, clearly stunned by the news.*)

REACTIONS TO DIAGNOSIS

Fred: (*Coming forward.*) It was kind of tough, you know. I mean, I guess I always thought there was a possibility. But when you actually hear the word cancer, that's something else again. You think you're going to die tomorrow. But you don't. It's just hard to get your head around the fact that things have changed.

Miriam: When you first find out, you're on an emotional roller coaster—there's anger, disappointment, and depression. I did a lot of crying the first night.

Man 2 (Jack):

They tell you that you have cancer, and all of a sudden your mind goes blank, and you don't hear what else is being said.

Woman 2 (Susan):

It was total disbelief. I'm too young for this. He's worked hard all his life, and now the kids are almost out the door, and we can finally look forward to some real quality time together, and this happens.

Jack: I left the doctor's office, drove to the liquor store, bought two bottles of brandy, swore a lot, got home about four, and by six, I couldn't stand up any more, and Susan had to carry me to bed (*chuckling*).

Susan: Not funny!

Man 3:   I've had a really hard time. I couldn't bring myself to tell my wife on the phone. I wasn't ready. So I waited until she got home that night. Margaret's reaction surprised me. She was aloof. What I needed was a hug and a kiss, which I eventually got, but I had to ask for it.

Jack: Homer Simpson is my favorite. Homer drank some radioactive stuff at his work, and the doctor says, well, you've got a pretty short time to live, and people in this situation go through four or five emotions. First of all, there's going to be disbelief, and denial—and grief—and anger, and finally acceptance. Homer says, "Ah, you've got the wrong guy." And then he goes: "I'm angrier than hell." Then he breaks down and cries for a while, and then he says, "Was that the last one? Oh, yeah," he says, "acceptance. Oh well, we'll get around to it some day." That's pretty funny. And I found I went through almost the same things.

Fred: You just wish the whole thing was a bad dream. (*Everyone exits but Miriam.*)

Miriam: I'm at such a loss. You'd think after 45 years of marriage I'd know what to do, but I don't. I love my Fred. And I know he's hurting. I can see that he's anxious, but he won't share it with me. I feel so shut out. How can I support him if he won't tell me what he's feeling? I know he likes to deal with problems on his own. I've learned to accept that. And maybe he can handle this illness best by not talking about it. But can he really? How can I tell? If I try to make him talk about his feelings, maybe it will make things worse. I just don't want him to have to deal with this alone. And I don't want to be alone with all my fears either. Could you make it all go away?

Bomb explodes, and actors scurry from the stage.

BATTLE SCENE

Woman 1:   (*Speaking directly in ear of Man 1, who is adjusting his army gear, but becomes increasingly frightened as* *he listens.*) So are you prepared to fight? Everything all right? Are you scared? Because if you are, it might be good for you to talk about it. I mean, it is a formidable enemy, really ruthless if it gets a good hold on you. You might die. Or you might be badly wounded. So feel free to talk about your fears. It'll make me feel better, too, to know what you're thinking. I can share the experience with you. Okay? Won't that be good?

FAMILY AND PERSONAL DYNAMICS

Three men are standing parallel to each other at a golf driving range, intermittently hitting balls. Two women are in the clubhouse, drinks in hand, chatting with each other. Women freeze while men talk; men freeze while women talk.

Man 3:   I'm not emotionally disturbed by any of this. It'll work out fine.

Man 2:   It hasn't really upset me at all.

Man 1:   I wasn't devastated. My wife was the one who was shocked.

Woman 1:   Fred refused to eat after he was told. It was two weeks before he'd eat something.

Woman 2:   Jack's trying to act as if he's not worried so that I'll feel better about it. But he does want me to know how to access all his bank accounts all of a sudden. Just in case. What does that tell you?

Man 2:   We didn't react very much, other than the first few minutes.

Man 3: It's not that big a deal.

Man 1: I'm actually more worried about my wife than I am for myself.

Woman 1: I told him that maybe I should learn to be more independent. You know, learn how to do the pilot light and all the things he looks after.

Man 2: I quickly came to terms with it. I only really got upset once, and that's when I called my brother.

Man 1: I keep telling my wife there's no sense worrying about something unless you can change it.

Woman 1: My one fear is that it's spread, but I don't say anything about that. The rest of it I can handle.

Man 1: There isn't a hell of a lot to talk about, to tell the truth.

Woman 1: He started breaking out in a cold sweat at night, so I knew he was worried. But "I'm fine, I'm fine. I'm dealing with it," he says. But he didn't sleep. He had bad dreams all night. He wasn't coping.

Man 2: If Susan were in a crisis, she'd talk about it to death—getting all worked up and emotionally strung out with this scenario and that. It's not that I won't talk about things; I just don't go on and on about it.

Woman 2: I know he's keeping things inside. I wish he'd spit it out. If I have to wonder why he's being silent, I'll start getting tense and bitchy.

Man 3: Previously Margaret and I talked about everything.

Like we've been married over ten years, and this seems to be the first thing that we really aren't talking about—I don't know what it is—fear on her part, or what?

Woman 2: He's probably too terrified to talk about it.

Man 2: (*Forcefully.*) I've told people that I will discuss it with them once. But it's not going to be the focal point of my life. I am not running away from it. I just think there are better things to talk about.

Man 3: She doesn't want to hear the bad news. It upsets her. So here I am at the stage where not only do I have to deal with the bad news, but I have to deal with her having to deal with it.

Man 1: Miriam has her own problems, and I don't want to add to those. And she's handling this really well, very positively. She's fine. (*Men 2 and 3 exit.*)

Woman 1: I think he feels that I don't need any support. He thinks this is his problem. His cancer. And he's the one who's facing all the problems and suffering (*starting to cry*). Well, he knows that there's a support group for wives at the Prostate Group, but I don't think Fred's ever sat back and figured out why wives need support. I don't think he figures there's any impact on me at all.

Man 1: I never believed that I should come home and dump my concerns. I was a foreman on my job, and had all this turmoil going on. If I came home and said to her that I had a problem with Bill, let's say, then she'd be at me going, "Who? Why is he doing that? Has he done it before? What did you say? What did he say? What are you going to do about it?" So I don't even want to go there. Women are different than men. They like details.

Woman 2:   I could use a large bottle of tranquilizers.

Man 2:   (*Striding to center stage, asking the audience.*) What are the four most threatening words a woman can say to a man?

Woman 2:   (*Approaching Man 2.*) We need to talk. (*Man 2 flees the stage followed in close pursuit by Woman 2.*)

COMPLICATED TREATMENT CONSIDERATIONS

Man 3 (Professor Joker):

(S*peaking rapidly, making wild gestures.*) There are some things you need to know about the treatment of prostate cancer. You could just decide to watch it and see what happens. Or you could have surgery, maybe nerve-sparing. And sometimes there's an option of having hormonal treatment before the surgery, or not. But you could also have radiation treatment, the traditional kind with an external beam. And you might want to consider conformal radiotherapy, or there are some hospitals where you can get radioactive seed implants, but you'll need to go on a waiting list. Then, of course, there is cryosurgery, although we're not so positive about that anymore. A better option may be microwave thermoablation, although that's only available in clinical trials. Down the road we'll be experimenting with more biological agents. We're not sure which approach is best, but there are advantages

and disadvantages with each one. Get some information, think about it, and go away.

GETTING INFORMATION

*Woman 1 throws colored paper cutouts in the air. When they land,
Woman 2 and Man 2 scurry around picking them up, repeating
"Information, Information." Then they try unsuccessfully to piece
them together like a jigsaw puzzle. Finally, in frustration, they both
exclaim in unison:*

Man 2 and Woman 2:
Information??!!

Man 3:   (*Comes forward, holding golf club in putting position.*) Prostate cancer is like golf: it's a lot more complicated than it seems at first glance. (*Exits.*)

Miriam and Fred sit together, facing the audience.

Miriam: It wasn't the easiest thing coming to a decision about
what to do. In the beginning the doctors and nurses
don't have time to sit with you and answer all your
questions.

Fred: Information is there but you have to go looking for it.
It's up to you.

Miriam: But there should be something set up for you in the
beginning when you're first told. Maybe not necessarily that very day because you're so scared. Maybe
the doctor should ask you to come back the next day
or a few days later to talk about it.

Fred: We went to the library …. (*Miriam interrupts.*)

Miriam: We got all sorts of pamphlets and books ….

Fred: (*Stopping Miriam.*) Yeah. Miriam read them to me every night in bed. Bedtime stories.

Miriam: And I talked to some friends whose husbands have been treated for prostate cancer. You hear all these horror stories….

Fred: (*Stopping her.*) In the end, we took the urologist's advice to go for the surgery.

Miriam: He gave us a lot of time and answered all our questions. Fred really liked him, didn't you, Fred?

Fred: Sure did. He sounds like he knows what he's talking about.

Miriam: But we wouldn't have been comfortable with our decision had we not done all that research on our own. (*Miriam and Fred exit.*)

Jack: (*Coming forward.*) Prostate cancer … what a joke. If you were expecting to get a straightforward solution to the problem, forget it. Each case is so individual. The "what ifs" can really stress you out. You know, there needs to be some psychological counseling for this operation. It's not like changing a headlight on a car. There are emotional repercussions with incontinence and impotence (*pause, then with more anger*). And Susan's the wrong one to talk with about it. She either gets too emotional or too protective, and I can't handle that right now. (*Jack exits.*)

UROLOGIST SCRUM

Woman 1 (Reporter):

Here come the urologists! (*Sticks her microphone in the face of one of the urologists.*) What about treatment for prostate cancer?

Man 3 (Urologist):

Treatments have major impact in terms of quality and quantity of life, and there are trade-offs between those two things. And the only way that a patient can make those decisions is to become educated. And it can be very difficult to get up to speed so that they're in a position to make the right decision for themselves.

Reporter: And do they get up to speed?

Man 3 (Urologist):

Well, they get up to *a* speed. I think most men can acquire enough of a sense of what the trade-offs are that they can make the right decision for themselves.

Woman 2 (Urologist):

With prostate cancer, there's so little definitive data— you tell them the pros and cons of all treatments, and they select. We really don't know what's best for them, as doctors, and I tell patients that.

Reporter: Isn't that unsettling for your patients?

Man 3 (Urologist):

We try to be reassuring, whatever the decision is.

Woman 2 (Urologist):

I tell them that they are not likely to die in a year or

two or five. I really try and hammer that in because I figure it gives them time to think about things and relax and make a better decision. I like well-informed, very realistic patients. I'm sorry; that's all the time we have for questions. (*Urologists start to exit, with reporter following them.*)

Reporter: But what about…. (*Exiting.*)

HOSPITAL SCENE WITH JACK AND FRED

In the background we hear a loudspeaker system. "Dr. Banerjee, please report to third floor, west wing…. Code Red, second floor east wing."

Two men walk onto the stage very painfully, and ease themselves onto adjacent chairs.

Jack: Don't I know you? I know … the golf course. I'm Jack. (*They shake hands.*)

Fred: Strange place to meet. I'm Fred. What are you in here for?

Jack: You know, the old waterworks.

Fred: Oh.

Jack: Prostate. It's gone now. They took it out. And you?

Fred: That's what I'm here for too.

Jack: Geez. It's an epidemic. They did mine three days ago. The first couple days were a bit rough, but I'm feeling better today. Say, have you had any problems with your catheter? Mine leaked a couple of times. (*Jack looks at Fred, but gets no response; his tone shifts to being deliberately cheerful.*) It's no big deal. I'm hoping to get out of here by tomorrow. Can't see why not.

Fred: That's the way to think about it. It's good to have a positive attitude. I'd like to get home, too.

Jack: Yep. I want to get back to work as soon as I can.

Fred: What do you do?

Jack: I'm in insurance. How about you?

Fred: Well, I'm semi-retired. But I keep my hand in doing a little real estate.

Jack: No kidding. Say, maybe I could get some advice sometime. My wife and I have been kicking around the idea of moving into a condo.

Fred: Sure, anytime. I'll get you a card from my room. (*Men start getting up from chairs; Jack puts a hand on Fred's arm.*)

Jack: Fred, that's quite a process, getting the catheter in, isn't it? A little uncomfortable.

Fred: (*Grimaces, showing that he finds this topic inappropriate.*) Oh, well, a little adversity is good for you, right? At least that's what my hockey coach used to tell us.

Jack: Yeah, I guess it's not much worse than getting a puck in the chops. Probably does make you stronger in the long run.

Fred: Toughens us up. Say, Jack, do you still play golf?

Jack: Every chance I get.

Fred: Maybe we could get together for a round sometime after we get out of here.

Jack: Sounds great.

Fred: In a couple of weeks or so?

Jack: If not sooner.

Fred: I'll go get you that card so we can keep in touch.

The two men hobble off, wincing in pain.

TELEVISION GAME SHOW

Man 3 (Game Show Host):

Welcome to "Slices of Life" (*encourages audience to clap*). Today we're asking the question: "Whom do you tell?" when you have cancer. We've got three couples to share their experience with us. Here's couple number one, Fred and Miriam. (*They come to center stage.*) Whom do you tell?

Miriam: Fred's not inclined to go telling everyone about his cancer. We told the family, his brothers, and our son especially. He felt they needed to know so they'd get tested, just in case. The most difficult was telling his mother; she's 90. We had to tell her because she'd be awfully hurt if she found out that we hadn't.

Fred: I don't mind saying to somebody, "Yes, I have prostate cancer." But I don't want sympathy. And to be truthful, I'm reluctant to tell the guys I work with because they usually joke around. Some of the younger guys say, "Ah, you old guys, you're impotent anyway."

Miriam: You never told me that.

Host: Thank you. Thank you (*escorting them offstage*).

Miriam: (*Talking as she exits.*) What a thing to say! Who said that? What did you say? Does that bother you? ...

Host: Now, we have couple number two, Susan and Jack. (*They come to center stage, holding hands and staring into the camera.*) Whom do you tell?

Susan: Having dealt with cancer in the family before, we decided that we didn't want a lot of people to know. We realized how focused the whole family can get on just the cancer. Of course we told the girls. They were shocked. They thought their dad was invincible. But they've been great, dropping by and phoning. Our eldest decided her dad needed to be in good shape for the operation, so she takes him off to the Y to do weights and swim together. And she even has us on an anti-cancer diet.

Jack: Yeah! No red meat and lots of broccoli. Anyway, I was pretty upfront at work. I mean, it's nothing to be ashamed of. I didn't do anything wrong to get this. I was going to be taking a lot of time off, so I told everyone during a staff meeting and said that if anyone had any questions they could feel free to talk to me. Well, I was a popular guy for a day. All the women wanted to know the details so that they could pass them on to their husbands. I think all the men in the office went right out and had their PSA tests done. Since I've been back to work, everyone's been really supportive. (*Couple exits.*)

Host: Thank you. And finally we have couple number three, Victor and Alice:

Man 1 (*now as Victor*):

(*Speaks in a gruff military voice.*) I don't see any point in making a big thing of it. It's no one else's business but ours. I told my wife not to tell anyone. I wouldn't like to be talked about, and I don't want to be seen as being weak. At work, I just told my colleagues I was going for an operation. After my operation, if people asked, I told them I had had cancer, but that I was cured. That shut them up.

Host: Thank you. (*Victor exits but Alice follows the host and tugs at his sleeve.*)

Alice: Maybe none of his friends know, but all mine do! But they've been sworn to secrecy. I needed some emotional support.

Host: Thank you (*trying to get rid of Alice*). Tune in next week when we ask the question, "How do you get what you need from your doctor?" (*Encourages audience to clap.*)

BATTLE SCENE

Woman 1:   This is quite a battle. Not what I was expecting at all.
How are you doing? Ready for another go? Are you
all right?

Man 1:   I need to talk. I'm really scared. What if we don't
make it? I'm not feeling very strong.

Woman 1:   Not strong?! Of course, you're strong! This is not the
time to talk about your feelings. You're making me
panic. Go back to being brave. PLEASE!

CONVALESCING

Woman 2 (Susan):

> (*Carrying laundry basket.*) It's very stressful. I want
all the wives to know that. If he's hurting, I'm hurting.
Sometimes I just don't know what to do for him. He
said he was in a lot of pain and had trouble peeing, but
I thought he was just uptight, so I tried to calm him
down instead of getting help. I totally misjudged the
situation. There was a blockage.

Woman 1:   (*Enters with coffee mug.*) He tries to tell me he's fine
all the time, that there's nothing wrong, that I worry
needlessly. When I ask him how he is today, "Oh, I'm
fine. I'm fine." And of course, he doesn't have to be
around me for five minutes for me to know perfectly
well that he's not fine. (*Women exit.*)

Man 3:   (*Coming to center stage.*) She never says anything
about what this is like for her, and, you know, I kind
of appreciate that.

Man 2:   (*Standing next to Man 3.*) It really is a crapshoot, you know. You have no idea what's ahead of you until after the surgery. Did they get all the cancer, or did it spread? You wonder if the incontinence will ever stop. You know you're totally impotent and feeling tender and in pain and wonder if it'll ever go away.

MEN'S INTERNAL VOICES

Man 1:   (*Facing out to audience, the other two men standing on each side looking at him.*) They were saying I'd need to take it easy for a little while, but I was up and down the stairs from the day I came home from hospital.

Man 2:   (*Shouting in Man 1's ear.*) You can take it.

Man 3:   (*Shouting in Man 1's ear.*) Give 'em hell. (*Men rotate.*)

Man 2:   (*Facing audience.*) I went back to work after six weeks. As a salesman I spend a lot of time in my car and that's creating problems up through my groin. They tell me it's because of the nerve damage from the operation. It's a big aggravation.

Man 3:   (*In Man 2's ear.*) Oh, poor baby.

Man 1:   (*In Man 2's ear.*) Having a rough time? (*Men rotate.*)

Man 3:   Here I am with cancer still left in my body, and nothing is being done. Are they waiting until it grows big again, and then they'll say, sorry, it can't be helped, you have to die? Or what?

Man 1:   (*In ear.*) Buck up.

Man 2:   (*In ear.*) Be a man. (*Men rotate.*)
Man 1:   I told my wife I wouldn't have any problems. She was
                  so worried I was setting myself up for disappointment
                  and depression. The day they removed the catheter, I
                  had control. No problems. And my wife had gone out
                  and collected bedpans and pads for the bed and dia-
                  pers in all shapes and sizes because she wanted us to
                  be prepared (*chuckles*).

Man 2:   (*In ear.*) Way to go.

Man 3:   (*In ear.*) You have to be strong. (*Men rotate.*)

Man 2:   I got up the Friday following the surgery and went to
                  work. I was only there four hours, and it was only half
                  days for a while. But I had to because if you sit at
                  home you soon start feeling sorry for yourself. And
                  once that begins you may find yourself in a depression
                  you can't get out of.

Man 3:   (*In ear.*) I'll give you something to cry about.

Man 1:   (*In ear.*) Big boys don't cry. (*Men rotate.*)

Man 3:   I was very surprised to find the cancer had gone into
                  the lymph nodes. I had felt we'd be out of the woods.
                  But it's not so. So I said, "Well, dear, we're going to
                  start doing the things we want to do now."

Man 2:   (*In ear.*) That's the fighting spirit.

Man 1:   (*In ear.*) That's the stuff. (*Men exit.*)

Woman 2:   When you're in pain you're self-absorbed. Sometimes he gets really critical. I've had to bite my tongue quite a few times.

Woman 1:   He was very short-tempered after the operation, very moody, which isn't like him at all. I really had to watch what I said. I could tell by looking at him he was in pain, but I didn't want to say every time, "How's the pain?" because he got tired of the question. (*Exits.*)

EARLY MORNING LAUNDRY

Woman 2 (Susan):

God knows why, but he started to insist on staying downstairs watching television until 1:30 or so in the morning, and we have an open concept home. And I'd say, "Turn it off; I've got to get some sleep." It was a really stressful time for me at work. And he said, "You can sleep. I'm not stopping you." He wouldn't listen. Well, it just so happened that I had two loads of laundry to do, so at 6 a.m., which is when I had to get up, I turned on the washer and dryer, which is right next to where he sleeps. There was no question of him sleeping in that morning. It was childish, I know.

THE GRUMPY BEAR SYNDROME

Man 3 (Professor Joker):

I'd just like to follow up on this point. Today we're going to demonstrate the Grumpy Bear Syndrome. This post-treatment syndrome is generally found in males, although it can be contagious when two people live in close quarters. The syndrome is characterized by: (1) periods of silent brooding, broken only occasionally by bear-like grunts; and (2) pronounced irritability. Our first example is a couple with fairly mild symptoms.

Woman 1 (Miriam):

I thought I heard you stirring. Here's your tea, dear.

Man 1 (Fred):

Hmm.

Miriam: Did you have a nice nap?

Fred: Mmm. Hmm.

Miriam: Freddie called to see how you were getting on.

Fred: Hmmm.

Miriam: He and Jill are going to drop by for lunch tomorrow. Won't that be nice? (*Fred sips his tea.*)

Fred: Tea's cold.

Miriam: All right, I'll get you another. (*Starts to leave.*)

Fred: I can do without.

Miriam: No, no, it's my fault (*martyred tone*). I should have brought it right up to you instead of putting in a load of laundry.

Fred: Miriam?

Miriam: (*Sounding exasperated.*) Yes?

Fred: I'm sorry. I do appreciate all that you're doing. It's just that I feel like such a lump.

Miriam: Well, I understand, dear (*moving over to hug him*). Just try to be a more cheerful lump.

Professor Joker:

Our next couple shows some of the more serious symptoms of the grumpy bear syndrome. They have reached the well-known "mollycoddling crisis point," which appears predictably at this high point in the irritability graph, about six to eight weeks post-treatment. Men are still relying on their wives for support but are also impatient to get back to normal. And women are starting to feel they're being taken for granted.

Jack starts to cross the stage, and Susan follows him.

Woman 2 (Susan):

Jack! Where are you going?

Man 2 (Jack):

We've got to get some wood in.

Susan: I don't need you to do that. That's all I need on top of everything, for you to get a hernia!

Jack: Well, we're low on wood.

Susan: I'll get some later. It's not like I'm loafing around, you know. I just haven't gotten around to it.

Jack: I'm perfectly capable of doing this. I'm fine now. (*Both are getting increasingly angry.*)

Susan: Sure you are. And I suppose you weren't tossing in
                your sleep moaning with pain last night.

Jack: I was not!

Susan: Oh, yeah? Well, tonight I'll record you.

Jack: (*Pointing his finger aggressively at Susan.*) You do
                that! But in the meantime stop hovering over me!

Susan: Fine! You want to do something useful—well, how
                about doing the dishes or folding the laundry? (*She
                throws laundry basket at him.*) I'm going to take the
                garbage out and shovel the snow. And then I'll split
                the wood.

Professor Joker:

                As you can see, this Grumpy Bear Syndrome can be
                very serious business. To help prevent things from
                getting really bad, our research team has compiled a
                list of **Eight Things to Do While Your Man is
                Recovering from Surgery ... Not!!!**

Actors line up across the stage.

Woman 1:   Every five minutes, ask how he's feeling or if he's in
                pain, morning to night.

Man 2:   If he says one revealing thing about what he's think-
                ing or feeling, immediately follow up by asking about
                the top five things you've always wanted him to open
                up about.

Woman 2:   Suggest that this might be a good time for him to retire,
                or give up smoking, or go on a diet, or take up yoga.

Man 1:   Invite all his friends and acquaintances around to the house for a bedside visit to help him overcome being such a stick in the mud.

Man 2:   Cancel the subscription to the television sports network.

Woman 1: Stay by his side at all times, and remind him to be careful every time he gets up from his chair.

Man 1:   While he's bed-ridden, use the opportunity to explain to him about steps that could be taken in your marriage to ensure a more equal distribution of power.

Woman 2: Let him get away with treating you like a servant or nursemaid. Some men ... okay, most men will use any excuse at all.

Professor Joker:
Oh, and then there's incontinence to deal with!

Everyone: GROAN!!

INCONTINENCE MESS

The actors move frantically around the stage, only stopping to speak their lines.

Man 2:   Now I know why babies cry when they're wet and soggy.

Man 1:   You don't know if you're going to go till you've gone.

Woman 1: It's pretty messy.

Man 3:   Lots of spillage.

Woman 2:   And the laundry!

Man 2:   It's embarrassing.

Man 3:   One amusing thing, though: you can sit at important meetings, piss your pants, and just smile. They haven't got a clue. (*Everyone laughs.*)

All exit except Man 1 who gets a golf club.

Man 1:   I don't have to wear pads anymore. The only time I'm in trouble now is when I'm drinking beer and playing golf at the same time. I can't do that. They didn't tell me that when they asked me to sign the informed consent for surgery. (*Exits.*)

ANOTHER UROLOGIST SCRUM

Man 3 (Reporter):

Here come the urologists! Can you shed some light on incontinence?

Woman 2 (Urologist):

It's one thing to think intellectually about the prospect of being incontinent and another to live with it day after day. It presents a whole series of challenges, and there can be a big impact on relationships.

Man 3 (Reporter):

What about erectile dysfunction?

Man 2 (Urologist):

> If the thought of being incontinent is a blow to self-esteem, the loss of sexuality—of erectile function—is a huge blow to a man's sense of being a man. The thought of dying, frankly, often becomes secondary to the quality of life issues that they have to address. Excuse me, I have patients waiting.

Reporter and female urologist freeze in scene while Man 2 crosses to other side of the stage to see his patient.

OFFICE VISIT

Man 2 (Urologist):

> (*Enters office where Fred and Miriam are waiting.*) Sorry, I had to do an interview. How are you, Fred?

Fred: Fine, and you? (*Miriam elbows Fred.*)

Urologist: (*Taken aback by the question.*) I'm fine. Now let's see (*looks at file*), we haven't discussed anything concerning sexual function.

Fred: Right (*very matter-of-fact*).

Urologist: What can you tell me about that?

Fred: I'm really not bothered about it.

Urologist: Have you had any erections?

Fred: No.

Urologist: Any sensations at all?

Fred: No.

Urologist: (*Closing the file.*) I know this can be hard to talk
                 about, Fred, but have you thought at all about any of
                 the techniques for helping with erections?

Fred: No.

Miriam: (*Leaning over Fred's shoulder.*) You were wondering
                 about Viagra, weren't you, Fred?

Fred: (*Looking uncomfortable.*) Yeah, I guess I was.

Urologist: Well, that's one possibility. But there are also mechan-
                 ical devices and injections to consider.

Fred: (*Even more uncomfortable.*) I don't know. What do
                 you think, Miriam?

Miriam: It's whatever you want, dear. But I think you might be
                 happier if we tried something. How about if I go feed
                 the parking meter and you and the doctor talk a bit
                 more about it?

Fred: (*Looking totally panicked.*) Okay.

Urologist: Fred, if you would just have a look at those pamphlets
                 beside you and think about any questions you might
                 have, I'll be right back.

*Urologist moves back into the scrum scene on opposite side of the
stage.*

Reporter: Doctor, do patients have trouble coping with erectile
                 dysfunction?

Man 2 (Urologist):

Most of them will tell you that sexuality is not a huge part of their relationship and, while that may be true in many cases, in others there may just be awkwardness in broaching the subject. I almost always have to bring up erectile dysfunction with my patients; they tend not to, which I find interesting.

Woman 2 (Urologist):

You can still have a good sex life with erectile dysfunction. All you need is playfulness, imagination, and a sense of humor.

Man 2 (Urologist):

(*Glaring at female urologist and rolling eyes together with reporter.*) Easy for you to say!

Man 2 and 3:

(*In unison.*) Women! They just don't get it!

Woman 2 (Urologist):

No more questions, please. (*She exits, two men remain.*)

Man 3: (*Speaking to Man 2.*) Sex is like hockey. You can make all kinds of fancy moves, but in the final analysis you want to put the puck in the net. (*They laugh and leave together.*)

Man 1: Sexual potency is not what makes you a man.

Man 2: I'd rather die than lose my potency.

Woman 2: I didn't realize getting an erection is so sacred to him.

Man 3:   It isn't a problem, really.

Man 2:   You begin to wonder whether you have any worth.

Woman 2:   I've tried to touch him, but he pulls away. I miss the tenderness.

Man 3:   Now we hug a lot more.

Woman 1:   We kind of stay away from that part of our life, because nothing happens, and all you do is get each other frustrated.

Man 1:   At least I don't have performance anxiety any more.

Woman 2:   I would be happy if suddenly he had some returning function and we could have sex again, but I'm not devastated that we don't have it. I'd rather live without sex and have my husband.

Man 2:   If other men knew I was incapable of a sexual relationship, they'd be sniffing around my wife. They wouldn't see it as a moral issue. They would see it as a feather in their cap.

Man 1:   We talk about it, joke about it, and treat it lightly. It's the easiest way.

Woman 1:   I'm not going to run away and find another husband.

Woman 2:   I can live without it.

Woman 1:   I can live without it.

Man 3:   I can live without it.

Man 1:   I can live without it.

Man 2 (Jack):

I really didn't expect to be impotent.

Other actors turn to stare at him, then leave the stage. Jack steps forward.

Jack: I chose the prostatectomy because I was told that without it I probably could expect ten good years, but with it I could look forward to double that. At the time it seemed like a good idea. Before the radiation I couldn't get an erection, but I could still experience orgasm. Now, I don't even have that. We tried injections, and they worked at first, but they don't any more. Nothing seems to work. I've become a eunuch. And if a man tells me he can deal with that, then he's lying. I wasn't prepared for this. I'm in my mid-50s, and I don't know how to be at peace with it. And no one wants to talk about the impact of impotence on your psyche. Am I really the only one who is having a hard time with this?

Miriam: Yes, it's hard to lose the sexuality. But we've been married 45 years, and our relationship is solid. If he had a heart attack and died, or an accident—that would be hard. But as long as he's here and we can still walk down the street together, or listen to music, or play with our grandchildren, or have tea and read the paper to each other—that's what's special.

Susan: This may sound nasty, but it's not really, but I feel that if he is impotent, maybe it'll slow him down. I just don't have as much desire any more. And I understand that happens to quite a few women my age. So if he can kind of slow down a bit, maybe it'll blend us out more evenly for our old age so that we can cope better. Because I just wonder, you know, after a couple of years, he may be dissatisfied with me. You know, find himself a younger woman or whatever. (*Bomb explodes, and actors flee the stage.*)

BATTLE SCENE

Man 1 and Woman 1 enter together, looking battle weary.

Man 1:   We've come a long way through this campaign. There've been some heavy losses though.

Woman 1:   It makes me sad.

Man 1:   Me too. Things will never be quite the same.

Woman 1:   That's true. But I'm thankful you're still here.

Man 1:   And I'm thankful you're still here. I couldn't have done it without you (*Bomb goes off, and they shrug and exit with resignation.*)

E.D. HOT LINE

Man 3:   (*Sprawling in chair. Phone rings and he answers.*) Good evening. ED hotline, Richard speaking. I see, it isn't working quickly enough for you. She fell asleep before anything started to happen. Oh well, tough luck. Say, did you hear about how Viagra and Disneyland are similar? Yeah, in both cases there's a one-hour wait for a three-minute ride. Well, excuse me. Aren't we touchy tonight?

Man 3: (*Answering phone again, now speaking with Spanish accent.*) ED hotline. Ricardo here. Yes, you'd like to know about non-standard approaches to sex. Your husband is too embarrassed to call himself. Isn't he the silly one? We'll send him a copy of our best seller, *Innovative Sexual Techniques for Dummies.* Don't mention it.

Man 3: (*Answering phone again, very business-like.*) ED hotline. Dick here. What's up? Uh huh. Doctor suggests you and the wife develop more playfulness in bed. You have ED. Married 35 years. And you and your wife have never talked about sex? (*Pause, then with glee.*) Well, it's too late to start now! (*Gets to his feet.*)

BARNUM AND BAILEY SEX AIDS SHOW

Man 3: Ladies and gentlemen, the latest technology to help you put a tiger in your tank, jet fuel in your rocket, and a banana in your pocket. First we have Viagra (*roll down banner with picture of pills*)—famous for the three-hour erection. The vacuum pump (*roll down banner with picture of bicycle pump*)—pump yourself to attention. And then there's injections (*roll down banner with picture of very long needle*)—helps if you're married to a nurse. Injections: the choice of couples with steady hands and nerves of steel.... (*Exits.*)

MISS MAKING LOVE TO MY WIFE

Fred: It's been more than a year now that I had the surgery.
                 And I have to admit that hope is fading that I'll ever
                 recover the sexual piece. I mean, there's this one guy
                 at the support group who had it come back almost two
                 years after his surgery. But my sense is that that's
                 pretty unusual. I don't want you to get me wrong here.
                 I'm grateful to be alive, to live in a country where I
                 could get treatment. And I have nothing but praise for
                 all the people at the hospital. My urologist was super.
                 And Miriam and I are so lucky, to still be in love after
                 all these years. Sure we've had our tough times. Who
                 hasn't? But she's my best friend. Every morning we
                 walk down through the woods there and look at
                 what's coming into bloom, that kind of thing. And
                 then we sit and drink our tea on the porch here and
                 read pieces of the paper to each other. Since I retired,
                 we'll often go and lie down in the middle of the day.
                 Before the surgery, we'd make love sometimes, but
                 now I'll just stroke her hair, and we'll hold each other,
                 and she'll chat and I'll listen. It's very precious. But
                 still, there are moments that I can hardly stand it, the
                 fact that we can't make love the way we used to. And
                 I think if Miriam wasn't so worried about hurting my
                 feelings, she'd say the same thing. But don't get me
                 wrong. We're not going to mope around. We have a
                 good life. And Miriam will always be the woman for
                 me.

                 I see my grandchildren and some are at the age where
                 they're obsessed with sex. But, you know, it's wasted
                 on them … (*chuckling*), just like it was wasted on me
                 when I was their age. (*Exits.*)

TEACHER MONOLOGUE

Man 3:   I've been given back my life. How could I even think of complaining? For shame! You know, I used to tell my students that, right now, the things that are paramount in your mind are money, cars, fancy clothes, and sex, but, believe it or not, some day other things will be more important. I mean, in the beginning the physical part of a relationship is pretty big stuff, nobody would underestimate the importance. But things change with time. We're at a point where we look back on a healthy relationship. We've had a pretty good go. And now it's time to enjoy other things. Maybe I'd feel differently if I were 35 or 40, but at this stage in my life it really is fine. You might not believe what I'm saying, but it's true. And my wife, she's just been my strength all the way along. I couldn't believe how important she has been, you know. So very important.

THE FUTURE – GETTING BACK TO LIVING

Susan: (*Holding laundry basket, shouting.*) Jack! Jack! What about the lawn mower? Are you going to put it away? It looks like rain. Jack! Jack! Oh, where is he? (*Goes off to find him, shouts from off stage.*) Jack!

Jack: (*Center stage.*) All right. All right, I can hear you. (*Addressing the audience.*) Ain't life grand! Six months ago I was getting the royal treatment. The object of loving concern because of that little blip in the system. Well, the blip's gone, at least for the time being, and it's back to "Jack, do this, Jack, do that" again. I wouldn't have it any other way. I mean, there's been loss, and there's uncertainty. And I know there will be tough times to come. But still, there's so much to life. So much to be positive about.

Susan: (*Offstage, and very loud.*) Jack!

Jack: Like that, for example. Music to my ears! (*Now shouting at Susan.*) Hold your horses, I'm coming! (*Exits.*)

BATTLE SCENE

Man 1:   I think the war might be over. Don't hear any sounds of battle anymore.

Woman 1:   So can we take these silly helmets off?

Man 1:   Yes, but keep them close by just in case. (*Both take helmets off.*) It might be just a cease-fire.

Woman 1:   I suppose.

Man 1:   You never know what might fall out of the sky.

Woman 1:   No matter what it is, I'll be right behind you—pushing you through it. (*He gives her a look.*) Just kidding! (*Soldiers exit arm in arm.*)

THE LAST WORD

Professor Joker:

Life is like golf and hockey. Run along now, and think about it.

RESEARCH-BASED THEATRE

I wrote the No Big Deal? *script together with my friend and colleague Vrenia Ivonoffski, artistic director of Act II Studio in Toronto. In developing the script we drew on the interview transcripts from our study of men with prostate cancer and their spouses.[1] Unlike the study on which all the narrative accounts in the book are based, the couples study was limited mostly to middle- and upper-class white men and their wives. Also, all of the men in the study were treated with a radical prostatectomy. Because of these limitations, we want to be careful and state here that* No Big Deal? *has probably not attended adequately to the possible variations in men's experiences across cultures and treatments. Nevertheless, we know from the enthusiastic reaction of many audiences that it has relevance for ill men.*

No Big Deal? *was performed for audiences of urologists, family physicians, health administrators, prisoners, factory workers, and, especially, members of prostate cancer support groups and their families and friends. The media became interested, and articles appeared in national, regional, and local newspapers. I was interviewed on national radio.[2] And excerpts from the play have been included in a documentary television program airing across Canada in 2002.*

No Big Deal? *was our second research-based drama. The first production we undertook, entitled* Handle with Care?, *was about the experiences of women with metastatic breast cancer. We wrote a story about that project,* Standing Ovation: Performing Social Science Research About Cancer.[3] *In the telling of the story, we described what we've learned about translating research findings into drama.*

If any reader decides he would like to round up some actors and take No Big Deal? *onto the stage, please contact me first for permission.*

We've made a VHS videotape of the No Big Deal? *drama. It can be ordered for $30 from the Psychosocial & Behavioural Research Unit, 790 Bay Street, Suite 950, Toronto, Ontario, Canada, M5G 1N8.*

REFERENCES

1. Gray, R. E., Fitch, M., Phillips, C., Labrecque, M., & Fergus, K. (2000). Managing the impact of illness: The experiences of men with prostate cancer and their spouses. *Journal of Health Psychology, 5*, 531-548.

2. Gray, R. E. (in press). Performing on and off the stage: The place(s) of performance in arts-based approaches to qualitative inquiry. *Qualitative Inquiry.*

3. Gray, R. E., & Sinding, C. (2002). *Standing ovation: Performing social science research about cancer.* Walnut Creek, CA: Altamira Press.

Appendix A

The prostate is a walnut-shaped gland that lies below the bladder. Among other functions, it mixes the components of ejaculatory fluid. As men hit age 40, the prostate starts to enlarge, and prostate problems occur. The vast majority of men experience a slowing of their urinary stream, a need to urinate more frequently, and more difficulty emptying the bladder. These symptoms can be expected and are not usually due to prostate cancer, unless they develop extremely rapidly.[1]

Some men have been shown to be at increased risk for prostate cancer. Men who are over age 60 are much more likely to be diagnosed than are younger men. Black men are more at risk than are Caucasian men, who in turn are more at risk than Asian men. Men with one or more close relatives diagnosed with prostate cancer are at higher risk of being diagnosed. And men on a high-fat diet are at greater risk than men on a low-fat diet.[2] Research into strategies to prevent prostate cancer suggest likely benefits from reducing fat intake, taking selenium and vitamin E supplements, and eating plenty of soybean products and cooked tomatoes.[1]

The purpose of screening is to identify prostate cancer at the earliest possible stage. The two main procedures are the digital rectal exam (DRE) and the prostate specific antigen (PSA) blood test. There are major controversies related to the benefits of these tests, especially PSA testing. Critics argue that raised PSA levels cause anxiety and necessitate biopsies that often do not lead to a diagnosis of prostate cancer. They also point out that some prostate cancers that are diagnosed might never have become clinically significant and necessary to treat—so that individual men may suffer treatment side effects for no good reason. Despite these (and other) concerns, PSA testing has been shown to be good at detecting clinically significant cancers (especially in conjunction with DRE), and there is mounting evidence that treatments prolong life following early diagnosis.[3]

Given all the scientific controversy surrounding screening for prostate cancer, it's understandable that expert groups and organizations are not in agreement. Most argue, however, that men should be fully informed of the pros and cons of screening so that they can be involved in deciding if they want to be tested.[3] Unfortunately, research with Canadian family physicians has revealed that discussions between men and their physicians about PSA testing rarely occur.[4]

About one in eight men in North America will be diagnosed with prostate cancer. When prostate cancer is diagnosed, it is classified along two dimensions: (1) grade (the intensity or aggressiveness of the cancer cells) and (2) stage (the extent of the spread of disease). This is information that a doctor should provide to patients, as it is critical for helping to decide on an appropriate treatment. While there is variability across prostate cancers, the majority of tumors are slow growing (low or intermediate grade), and most men will live at least ten years without any treatment.[5]

For cancer that is contained within the prostate there are three main treatment options: surgery (radical prostatectomy), radiation therapy (external beam or brachytherapy), and watchful waiting. Each has its advantages and disadvantages. While studies have found surgical patients tend to live longer, they also have the highest incidence of serious side effects (like urinary incontinence and erectile dysfunction).

External beam radiation is often used for cancer that has spread just beyond the walls of the prostate. But once the cancer has spread, other measures are often instituted. The main approach to treating prostate cancer that has spread to the lymph nodes or beyond (usually to the bones, but sometimes to the lungs or liver) is to reduce the level of testosterone and other adrenal male hormones. This can be accomplished through surgical or chemical castration. For the latter, there is a growing arsenal of drugs and ongoing experimentation with various combinations and schedules of administration of the drugs.[6]

Eventually hormone therapy ceases to slow the growth of cancer. While there remain a number of approaches for helping with quality of life, none of the additional treatments that have been evaluated has shown improvement in men's survival times.[1]

REFERENCES

1. Klotz, L. (2000). *Prostate cancer: A guide for patients.* Toronto: Prospero Books.

2. Gallagher, R. P., & Fleshner, N. (1998). Prostate cancer: Individual risk factors. *Canadian Medical Association Journal, 159,* 807-813.

3. Meyer, F., & Fradet, Y. (1998). Prostate cancer: Screening. *Canadian Medical Association Journal, 159,* 968-972.

4. Gray, R. E., Carroll, J., Goel, V., Orr, V., Fitch, M., Chart, P., Fleshner, N., Morris, B. A. P., & Greenberg, M. (1999). Canadian family physicians and prostate cancer: A national survey. *Canadian Journal of Urology, 6,* 892-897.

5. Nam, R. K., Jewett, M. A. S., & Krahn, M. D. (1998). Prostate cancer: Natural history. *Canadian Medical Association Journal, 159,* 685-691.

6. Gleave, M. E., Bruchovsky, N., Moore, M. J., & Venner, P. (1999). Prostate cancer: Treatment of advanced disease. *Canadian Medical Association Journal, 160,* 225-232.

Appendix B

REFLECTIONS ON THE WRITING OF *PROSTATE TALES*:
LOCATING THE WORK WITHIN PERSONAL AND ACADEMIC CONTEXTS

As I commented in the prologue, the style of *Prostate Tales* is not much like that of most research reports. Narrative accounts and dramatic scripts are not the standard vehicle for communicating researchers' understanding of social issues. Nevertheless, *Prostate Tales* is not unique, and my experimentation with non-standard writing fits within an exciting movement in the social sciences focused on finding new ways of representing research findings.[1,2] Laurel Richardson, one of the leaders in this movement, has argued that it is no longer even appropriate to think of the many new writing approaches as "alternative" to an accepted mainstream approach. She argues that the new writing approaches are in and of themselves valid and desirable representations of the social; they need not be constantly compared to a now suspect "standard" writing approach. Richardson coined a phrase to try and capture the positive aspects of these writing approaches—"Creative Analytic Practices."[1]

Why did this shift towards Creative Analytic Practices occur? In large part, it is an expression of a changed way of thinking in the social sciences about the nature of knowledge. In former days, it was possible for researchers to claim a kind of omniscient objectivity about their studies. If they followed pre-specified methods of data collection and reported their findings in particular linear and rational ways, then they could make claims to having unlocked the truth of a particular social issue. This position is no longer tenable given the many challenges that have been brought against it in the last few decades, most notably by theorists influenced by postmodernism.

These days, most social scientists accept, to greater and lesser degrees, that researchers are greatly implicated in the studies they do, that it is not possible for them to be ultimately objective, and that the methods they use (standard or not) and their ways of reporting inevitably shape knowledge. Postmodernism takes this further, fostering the doubt that any method or theory has a universal claim to being "right," that there is any possibility of ever assigning a straightforward "truth" to complex social matters. Postmodernism assumes that all styles and approaches to writing about research findings, as with the research process, are necessarily partial, local, and situational; they are never able to nail things down in any ultimate way.[1] A major implication of these changes in thinking about knowledge has been to open up the social sciences to considering all manner of approaches. Collectively, social scientists are engaged in "thinking outside of the box"—a box that has limited so much of our activity in the past. Creative Analytic Practices is a (perhaps *the*) wave of the future for the social sciences.

There is another influence on the trend to new writing and performance practices in the social sciences. Increasingly there is pressure from government funding agencies and university administrations for academics to demonstrate relevance of their work and to ensure that it has influence in the larger social context.[3] Historically, dissemination of research findings has been vastly undervalued within academia, with little system encouragement or support for individual scientists interested in communicating their results beyond the usual academic journals. The result has been that "knowledge" has tended to travel within tight circles of academics, having little currency among the people who have been studied or the wider society. I love Laurel Richardson's comments about this situation. "It seems foolish at best and narcissistic and wholly self-absorbed at worst, to spend months or years doing research that ends up not being read and not making a difference to anything but the author's career" (p. 517).[4] This has been the status quo. But more than ever before, the challenges of dissemination (and "knowledge translation") are being discussed, and there is new encouragement and openness about approaches that address the challenges. Our work with research-based theatre is a good example. I think that a decade ago it would have been virtually impossible to find funding for such an "outside-of-the-box" approach. But there has been enormous interest in our work, from cancer educators, health professionals and policymakers, researchers, and community organizations. Clearly, it is an opportune time in history for researchers interested in developing effective Creative Analytic Practices.

With these shifts in the social sciences towards new approaches and forms, there has been a flurry of activity aimed at defining criteria for judging such work. Old ways of assessing research reports have dubious relevance for Creative Analytic Practices like *Prostate Tales*. In what follows, I will draw upon the writings of several commentators concerned with evaluative criteria as I consider the *Prostate Tales* project.

There is agreement among commentators that researchers/writers should be present in their texts through an explicit self-accounting and should also be implied and felt throughout their texts.[1,5,6] I've struggled with this expectation, fearing that too much of my own presence in the accounts would draw away from the main characters—men with prostate cancer. I also anticipated that my main readership would likely not be academics keen to see evidence of self-reflexivity at every turn. More likely, men with prostate cancer and others connected to them are my main readers. My guess is that they are more interested in the accounts and less in the process I've gone through in constructing them. Given these concerns, I've decided to remain largely absent through the text, addressing aspects of my engagement with the prologue in the preface and particularly in this appendix.

One aspect of self-reflexivity involves explicating the process that has been involved in my writing of the text. In revealing this process I also address the expectations articulated by Cole and Knowles—that researchers use a principled process, attempt procedural harmony in their writing, and be internally consistent in their approach.[5] At one point in this project I considered going through and detailing the decisions I made with each of the accounts, so as to make transparent the principles that guided my writing. Instead of such an intensive approach, let me offer a simple example, "Carl Retreats to the Den." This account was based primarily on one man's interviews. I had originally read his transcripts as part of our research team's analysis of the interviews gathered for our in-depth study of prostate cancer and masculinity. I looked at the notes that I'd made from those earlier discussions, remembering what various team members had seen as particularly illuminating or interesting in the transcripts. Then I read the transcripts again, re-making a list of the key issues. I looked for what moved me most emotionally. After considerable reflection, I made a decision to focus the story on the marital relationship and also to reveal some of the race-related issues that were so profoundly displayed in this man's transcripts. Although this decision was linked to what I had read in the transcripts (and how I was affected by what I read) and to comments from research team members, it was also influenced by my overall sense of the evolving manuscript. I considered the number and variety of issues that I had covered or would be covering in the other accounts, making sure that there would not be too much duplication. For example, in "Carl Retreats to the Den," I didn't go into great detail about interactions with doctors because I had focused almost exclusively on that aspect in another account. With this narrative account, as with others, I made decisions to leave pieces of this man's life out, or gave them secondary importance. For example, I revealed the importance of religious beliefs but didn't make it a centerpiece of the story (I could have written a quite different account that focused on the rich connections between illness and religious life). I created a rough plot line. I compiled direct quotes that were particularly relevant to the key issues and imagined scenes that were suggested from his interviews. I wrote a draft of the account. In this draft, I deliberately went beyond the obvious, drawing on suggestions (however slight) that were present in the interviews to highlight the character's emotional reactions and internal thoughts. Then I looked at the transcripts from several of the other men in our study, looking for pieces relevant to the main issues of "Carl's" account, details that could be included to elaborate the issues and to help disguise the identity of the story's primary teller. I revised the account, adding the details I'd selected from other men's experiences and altering any identifying information.

The process I went through in writing "Carl Retreats to the Den" shows the main steps I took in my process of writing narrative accounts, although there was certainly variability in this process across stories. The process for developing *No Big Deal?*, the drama we performed live for audiences, was quite different. In collaboration with Vrenia Ivonoffski, I pulled together a group of men with prostate cancer and their spouses, researchers, and volunteer actors. Together we read and discussed interview transcripts from our longitudinal study of couples dealing with prostate cancer. The men with prostate cancer spoke about their personal experiences, allowing an entryway for the others to their experiences. Then Vrenia guided us through countless improvisation exercises, pursuing deeper understandings of the major themes of the research. In the end, we had a menu of quotations from interview transcripts, stories from participants in the script development group, and images and scenes from the improvisation exercises. Vrenia and I went away and wrote a script. After we'd completed a draft, we performed it for trial audiences of prostate cancer patients, health professionals, and theatre experts. We revised the script and kept revising until we were satisfied. Then we took the production on tour.[7]

In the above descriptions of the processes of creating narrative accounts and dramas, it should be clear to the reader that there are many judgment points along the way and that authors make deliberate choices about what to include and what not to include. Narrative accounts reflect the analytic preferences of writers. This is to be expected, and it only becomes a problem when choices are not linked to clear intellectual and moral intentions.[5]

In beginning this writing project, I intended for *Prostate Tales* to help reveal the complex challenges facing men with prostate cancer, including the ways in which socially constructed notions of masculinity, personal relationships, and social and health systems/institutions influence how they are able to deal with illness. I wanted to make the struggles and triumphs of men with prostate cancer more visible to men themselves and more understandable to others. I did not want to tell romantic stories of heroism or victimization that would seek to draw emotions unnaturally out of unsuspecting readers. Rather, I wanted to tell stories that felt true, that honored the courage, humor and strength of individual men, while not hiding from everyday realities like fear, depression, and confusion. I sought to portray men's experiences authentically.

I undertook *Prostate Tales* believing that men with prostate cancer would find it useful to relate their personal experiences to those of the men in my accounts. I thought that the fictionalizing of the accounts would allow greater revelation of men's internal struggles than would usually be apparent in interactions they might have at a cancer support group or through an Internet discussion list—and that this greater revelation would be useful for men. Perhaps they might feel less alone with their situations and more likely to act on behalf of themselves and other men. I also hoped that family and friends and health professionals might better understand the dilemmas of men with prostate cancer and work to help where they can. Whether *Prostate Tales* makes the kind of "substantive contribution" that commentators feel should be expected of Creative Analytic Practices will depend in large part upon how well I've translated my intention into appropriate action.

A related criterion for a successful text is whether it is linked to social and political issues and able to stimulate action in the world.[5,6,8] Men's health issues have had little explicit attention until recently, and this has had important consequences. Too many men get inadequate assistance in making decisions. Some get inadequate medical attention. The people around them, often including health professionals, poorly understand how to be helpful. *Prostate Tales* does not provide solutions for these problems. But in undertaking this project, I intended to provide a window onto the particular challenges and dilemmas for ill men. The assumption beyond this strategy is that people will be more willing and more able to try to respond adequately when they fully appreciate what others are facing.

Some criteria for successful Creative Analytic Practices relate to how well texts are written.[8] Are characters well developed? Does the plot follow smoothly? Is the account pleasing to read? Does it move the reader emotionally? My intention has certainly been to provide accounts that are not just informational but evocative, compelling, and aesthetically pleasing. But readers must make their own judgments.

A related criterion is that accounts should provide abundant concrete detail, so that they express a sense of the everydayness of lived reality.[6,8] In writing *Prostate Tales*, I tried to provide detailed, "thick" descriptions of the situations, emotions, and relationships experienced by various men with prostate cancer. The accounts will hopefully provide readers with a strong sense of what it might be like to be inside these various men's lives. I hope that readers gain insights into particular experiences such as unemployment, marital discord, depression, incontinence, rage, erectile dysfunction, loss of libido, health system breakdown, communication difficulties, and so on. By providing stories from so many different men's perspectives, I hope to emphasize that there is not a single prostate cancer experience, but rather a multiplicity of experiences.[5,9] I hope that the cumulative experience of reading all the accounts prompts a visceral connection to the social realities of prostate cancer.

Carolyn Ellis writes that when she evaluates the success of a story she asks herself whether the writing has encouraged compassion for the main character(s).[8] This criterion speaks to the heart of my engagement with *Prostate Tales*. Indeed, chief among my goals with this writing has been to facilitate such compassion for men with prostate cancer—not just that others might feel compassion for ill men but that men might feel compassion for each other and for themselves. This has not been an easy undertaking, because I am very aware of how dangerously close compassion can be to pity and of how most men abhor the possibility of being pitied. My challenge as writer has been to steer clear of sentimentality and to portray men's experiences directly and honestly. If this has been done well, compassion will be possible—perhaps even inevitable.

REFERENCES

1. Richardson, L. (2000). New writing practices in qualitative research. *Sociology of Sport Journal, 17,* 5-20.

2. Denzin, N. (1997). *Interpretive ethnography: Ethnographic practices for the 21st century.* Thousand Oaks, CA: Sage.

3. Gray, R. E., Ivonoffski, V., & Sinding, C. (2001). Making a mess and spreading it around: Articulation of an approach to research-based theatre. In A. Bochner & C. Ellis (Eds.), *Ethnographically speaking* (pp. 57-75). Walnut Creek, CA: Altamira Press.

4. Richardson, L. (1994). Writing: A method of inquiry. In K. Denzin & Y. Lincoln (Eds.), *Handbook of qualitative research* (pp. 516-529). Thousand Oaks, CA: Sage.

5. Cole, A. L., & Knowles, J. G. (2001). Qualities of inquiry: Process, form and "goodness." In L. Neilsen, A. L. Cole, & J. G. Knowles (Eds.), *The art of writing inquiry* (pp. 211-219). Halifax, Nova Scotia: Backalong Books.

6. Bochner, A. P. (2000). Criteria against ourselves. *Qualitative Inquiry, 6,* 266-272.

7. Gray, R. E., & Sinding, C. (2002). *Standing ovation: Performing social science research about cancer.* Walnut Creek, CA: Altamira Press.

8. Ellis, C. (2000). Creating criteria: An ethnographic short story. *Qualitative Inquiry, 6,* 273-277.

9. Denzin, N. (2000). Aesthetics and the practices of qualitative inquiry. *Qualitative Inquiry, 6,* 256-265.

Glossary

ANALGESICS: Drugs used to kill pain. See "I Was Just a Number," "Darren Celebrates a Birthday."

BIOPSY: An approximately 20-minute procedure in which a needle "gun" is used to remove tissue samples from the prostate gland. See "Roger Discovers His Prostate," "Jed Meets Brad and Steven."

BRACHYTHERAPY: Putting tiny radioactive "seeds" or "tubes" inside the prostate gland where there's evidence of cancerous tissue. See "Carl Retreats to the Den," *No Big Deal?*.

CHEMOTHERAPY: Using drugs to kill cancer cells. See "Darren Celebrates a Birthday."

CLINICAL DEPRESSION: Feeling low, hopeless, blue, and/or down in the dumps for a few weeks, and losing interest in just about everything. Other common symptoms include changes in appetite, sleep problems, loss of energy, feelings of worthlessness, indecisiveness, and preoccupations with death or suicide. See "Jed Meets Brad and Steven," "Doug Goes Fishing," "I Was Just a Number."

CONFORMAL RADIOTHERAPY: Through use of computer technology, radiation can be more precisely targeted to just the prostate gland (and not surrounding area). This approach allows for higher doses of radiation to be delivered to the cancerous area. See "Maurice Runs a Meeting," *No Big Deal?*.

CRYOSURGERY: Using freezing to destroy cancer cells. See *No Big Deal?*.

DIGITAL RECTAL EXAM: The doctor inserts his finger in a man's anus and feels the prostate for any abnormalities. See "Roger Discovers His Prostate," *No Big Deal?*.

ERECTILE DYSFUNCTION: Problems related to a man getting and keeping an erection. See "I'll Sail Away," "Maurice Runs a Meeting," "Jed Meets Brad and Steven," "Ben Answers the Phone," "John Takes a Walk," "Norm Downs a Few Drinks," "Doug Goes Fishing," "I Was Just a Number," "Simon Cultivates Romance," *No Big Deal?*.

EXTERNAL BEAM RADIATION THERAPY: Using x-rays to kill cancer cells. See "I'll Sail Away," "Maurice Runs a Meeting," "Carl Retreats to the Den," "Jed Meets Brad and Steven," "Norm Downs a Few Drinks," "Simon Cultivates Romance," "Darren Celebrates a Birthday," *No Big Deal?*.

GLEASON SCORE: A grading system for cancer cells, out of ten, where higher scores indicate more aggressive cancer. See *No Big Deal?*.

HORMONAL THERAPY: A variety of drugs, used alone or in combination, to drastically reduce the level of male hormones in a man's body. See "Maurice Runs a Meeting," "Jed Meets Brad and Steven," "Simon Cultivates Romance," "Darren Celebrates a Birthday," *No Big Deal?*.

HORMONE REFRACTORY DISEASE: Prostate cancer that no longer responds to hormone therapy. See "Darren Celebrates a Birthday."

HOT FLASHES: Waves of bodily heat that are a side effect of hormone therapy. See "Jed Meets Brad and Steven," "Simon Cultivates Romance."

IMPOTENCE: Problems related to a man getting and keeping an erection. Now referred to as erectile dysfunction. See "I'll Sail Away," "Maurice Runs a Meeting," "Jed Meets Brad and Steven," "Ben Answers the Phone," "John Takes a Walk," "Norm Downs a Few Drinks," "Doug Goes Fishing," "I Was Just a Number," "Simon Cultivates Romance," *No Big Deal?*.

LIBIDO: The desire to have sex. See "Simon Cultivates Romance."

METASTASES: Cancer cells that have spread beyond the original site (e.g., prostate gland) to other parts of the body (e.g., bones). See "Jed Meets Brad and Steven," "Simon Cultivates Romance," "Darren Celebrates a Birthday."

MICROWAVE THERMOABLATION: Using heat to kill cancer cells. See *No Big Deal?*.

PALLIATION: Treatment when a man's life span is short; usually focused on controlling symptoms and maximizing comfort. See "Darren Celebrates a Birthday."

PC-SPES: A combination of seven Chinese herbs plus one North American herb (Saw Palmetto). PC-SPES has recently been withdrawn from the North American market because of reported impurities in the mixture. See "Maurice Runs a Meeting."

PENILE PROSTHESIS: A treatment for erectile dysfunction, usually used when other approaches have failed. A device is surgically implanted into the penis, and it can be inflated to achieve erection when a man wishes. See "Simon Cultivates Romance."

PROSTATE SPECIFIC ANTIGEN (PSA) TEST: A blood test that measures the level of an enzyme produced by the prostate. Higher levels indicate increased likelihood of prostate cancer. See "Roger Discovers His Prostate," "Maurice Runs a Meeting," "Jed Meets Brad and Steven," "Simon Cultivates Romance," *No Big Deal?*.

RADICAL PROSTATECTOMY: Using surgery to remove the prostate gland. See "Roger Discovers His Prostate," "Maurice Runs a Meeting," "Jed Meets Brad and Steven," "Ben Answers the Phone," "John Takes a Walk," "Frederick Tries for a Job," "Norm Downs a Few Drinks," "Doug Goes Fishing," "I Was Just a Number," "Simon Cultivates Romance," *No Big Deal?*.

SCREENING: Using the PSA blood test and/or the digital rectal exam to look for indications of prostate cancer. See "Roger Discovers His Prostate."

SEED IMPLANT RADIATION THERAPY: Putting tiny radioactive "seeds" or "tubes" inside the prostate gland where there's evidence of cancerous tissue. Also called "brachytherapy." See "Carl Retreats to the Den," *No Big Deal?*.

SPHINCTER: A ring-like muscle that acts as a valve. Sometimes the urinary sphincter is surgically replaced to help deal with serious urinary incontinence. See "Urinary Incontinence."

STRESS INCONTINENCE: Urinating or peeing due to physical conditions (e.g., sneezing) that cause a rise in abdominal pressure. See "I Was Just a Number."

TESTOSTERONE: The primary male hormone, drastically reduced in men's bodies through hormone therapy. See "Simon Cultivates Romance."

TRANSURETHRAL SUPPOSITORIES: A treatment for erectile

dysfunction. A small tube is inserted into the hole at the tip of the penis (urethra) and drugs released. See "Erectile Dysfunction (Impotence)."

TUMOR: An abnormal growth, that may or may not be cancerous. See "Roger Discovers His Prostate."

URINARY INCONTINENCE: Urinating or peeing when you don't want to. See "Maurice Runs a Meeting," "Jed Meets Brad and Steven," "John Takes a Walk," "Frederick Tries for a Job," *No Big Deal?*.

VACUUM PUMP: A treatment for erectile dysfunction. A cylinder is placed over the penis. A vacuum is created around the penis, causing blood to flow in. Once the penis is erect a ring is placed around the base to maintain it. See "Maurice Runs a Meeting," "Simon Cultivates Romance."

WATCHFUL WAITING: Not treating the prostate cancer, but monitoring its growth with periodic blood tests and clinical assessments—so as to assess if and when treatment may be warranted. See "Maurice Runs a Meeting," "Jed Meets Brad and Steven," "Ben Answers the Phone," *No Big Deal?*.

Selected Resources*

Prostate Cancer Information:

American Cancer Society
http://www.cancer.org/
The largest cancer organization in the U.S. offers informative and comprehensive information about all kinds of cancer. The "All about Prostate Cancer" section of the website has detailed and overview guides on various issues. In addition, patients, their families, and the general public can call a 24-hour toll-free telephone information service at 1-800-ACS-2345.

Canadian Cancer Society
http://www.cancer.ca/
This is a national community-based organization of volunteers. The website features a detailed community service database for people seeking support locally, a cancer-related glossary with cancer-related terms, and other up-to-date cancer information.

Cancernet
http://cancernet.nci.nih.gov
The National Cancer Institute offers information on a range of topics related to prostate cancer including clinical trials, screening and statistics. Material is continuously reviewed and revised by oncology experts.

Cancer Information Service (U.S.A.)
http://cis.nci.nih.gov/
This is a free public service of the National Cancer Institute that aims to communicate and interpret research findings for the public in a clear and understandable manner. Current scientific findings are described on the website and there is also a toll-free telephone service where research findings can be discussed or questions answered. Toll-free number, 1-800-332-8615.

Cancer Information Service (Canada)
http://cis.nci.nih.gov/resources/intlist.htm
The Canadian Cancer Society has a toll-free telephone information service to provide Canadian residents access to the latest cancer information. Trained professionals answer questions on a wide range of topics. Contact information is also available for local programs and support services.
1-888-939-3333 (English or French)
1-888-261-4673 (Northern Aboriginal Languages)

Oncology.com
http://www.oncology.com
Medical experts review all medical content on this online resource that provides information on a range of cancer-related issues.

Cancer Patient Organizations:

Us Too International
http://www.ustoo.com
This support group organization is for patients affected by prostate cancer and their families. There are more than 500 chapters in the United States, Canada, Australia and Europe. Support groups offer peer counseling, education about treatment options, and discussion of medical alternatives. Contact information for local groups is found here, and there are links to other online support and informa-

tion resources. Us Too International can be reached toll-free at
800-80-USTOO (800-808-7866).

Man to Man (U.S.A.)
1-800-ACS-2345
This support program with the American Cancer Society offers
community-based group education, discussion, and support groups
for men with prostate cancer. Contact information for local programs is available by calling toll-free 1-800-ACS-2345. Some support groups may also invite wives and partners to attend meetings.
In other locations, wives and partners may meet separately in a
group known as side-by-side.

The National Prostate Cancer Coalition (U.S.)
http://www.pcacoalition.org
This organization is dedicated to bringing together and representing the interests of multiple organizations and individuals with an
interest in the prevention and cure of prostate cancer. Most U.S.
support groups are represented within the coalition.

Canadian Prostate Cancer Network
http://www.cpcn.org
This organization offers contact information for support groups
across Canada and online links to an extensive list of online
resources about prostate cancer. Information includes selected
archived material on prostate cancer and newsletters from support
groups across the country.

The National Coalition for Cancer Survivorship
http://www.canceradvocacy.org
This is a patient-led advocacy organization that gives voice to cancer survivors. Events, news, publications, programs, information,
resources and seminars are listed for people with all types of cancer. An online tour guide has been made available for use from

this site to guide new Internet users to credible sources of cancer information and resources.

Scottish Association of Prostate Cancer Support Groups
http://www.pcansupportscot.f9.co.uk/
This is an organization where support can be obtained online. Contact information is listed for the network of support groups throughout Scotland. Basic and detailed information on prostate cancer can be accessed at this site.

Prostate Help Association
http://www.personal.u-net.com/~pha
The general public in the United Kingdom can find information about prostate cancer from this organization. A support network of men willing to share their experiences with others can be accessed through this organization as well as many links to additional online resources about prostate cancer.

The Prostate Cancer Charity
http://prostate-cancer.org.uk
This charity provides support and information through a telephone help line, an online chat room and online message boards. There is a long exhaustive list of additional information and support resources related to prostate cancer at this site.

Foundations/Charities:

American Cancer Society
http://www.cancer.org/

Canadian Cancer Society
http://www.cancer.ca/

The Canadian Prostate Cancer Research Foundation
http://www.prostatecancer.on.ca
The primary goals of this charitable organization are to help men by
funding research that will lead to advances in screening, diagnosis
and treatment for prostate cancer. The organization also funds
research leading to long-term solutions to cancer such as prevention.

American Foundation for Urologic Disease
http://www.afud.org
This organization supports patient education, public awareness,
research, and advocacy towards the prevention and cure of uro-
logic disease. It sponsors a toll-free information line that receives
5,000 phone calls each month. The organization also funds
research and public education initiatives and publishes *Family
Urology*.

CaP Cure (Association for the Cure of Cancer of the Prostate)
http://www.capcure.org
This organization seeks private funding for prostate cancer
research. Collaboration between cancer survivors, scientists, and
advocates is sought in most projects to rapidly translate research
findings into treatments and cures.

The Prostate Cancer Charity
http://prostate-cancer.org.uk

* All websites listed herein were current as of September 22, 2002.

About the Author

Ross E. Gray, the co-director of the Psychosocial and Behavioral Research Unit, Toronto Sunnybrook Regional Cancer Center, has worked with cancer patients since 1987. He is widely published with more than 50 papers dealing with cancer-related issues. He is also co-author of two dramatic scripts about cancer-related issues. One of his plays, *No Big Deal?*, is currently being seen in Canada with a move to the United States in the near future. Gray is the primary investigator for six funded studies related to issues facing men with prostate cancer and their families and friends.

Legacy: A Conversation with Dad

by Ross E. Gray & Claire M. Gray

Legacy: A Conversation with Dad is a meditation on manhood, written as a father-son dialogue. The father's voice enters through excerpts from an unpublished autobiographical novel he wrote in the early 1960s, a few years before his death. The son, a social scientist, belatedly interacts with his father, reflecting on their separate and interconnected paths. In elaborating the theme of men's lives and masculinity, the son brings personal, professional, and academic perspectives to bear. He discusses his relationships with his father and other men, as well as his experiences as a psychologist working with ill men. He weaves the academic literature about masculinity throughout. The intensely personal is linked to broad social issues, illuminating dilemmas facing men today.

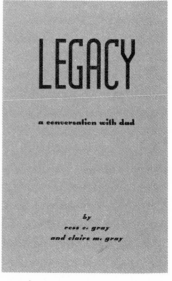

"Ross Gray takes us on a courageous and insightful journey into the shadows of his past. Through conversations with his deceased father, Gray offers insight into man's complex roles as father, friend, son, and lover. His compelling story of a son's endeavor to step out of his father's shadow enriches us and reveals truths about our own struggles to be free. Legacy *is an intensely open and intimate look into masculinity. Truly a book with heart!"*

Jim Bedard, Author of *Lotus in the Fire: The Healing Power of Zen*

*"*Legacy *is an honest, courageous, and sometimes painful self-reflection on the powerful imprint of a father who suffered from depression and committed suicide. Exploring his father's life through excerpts from his unpublished novel creates the unique format of father-son dialogue. The themes around masculinity touch common chords that ring clearly through the common life experiences of father and son. The book offers no easy answers to these issues, but the clarity and depth of their description provides comfort to men who worry that they might be alone in facing these struggles."*

Glen Palm, Professor of Child and Family Studies,
St. Cloud State University (Minnesota) and editor of *Working with Fathers*

0-9671794-2-4 (pbk) • 152 pages • 4 pages of photos • $14.95 (USA) / $22.95 (Canada)

To order, contact:
Men's Studies Press, P.O. Box 32, Harriman, TN 37748 USA
423/369-2375 • Fax 423/369-1125
www.mensstudies.com/Legacy